The following herb blends are provided for informational purposes only. Nothing in this recipe guide is intended to substitute for the medical expertise and advice of your primary health care provider.

You should discuss any decisions about treatment or care with your health care provider. The information contained within this guide is believed to be accurate at the time of writing but research is being undertaken daily and new information, effects, or side effects may be discovered that conflict with the materials contained herein.

No product, service, or therapy is endorsed by the author, publisher, or other individual associated with the creation of this material. The reader should remember that the U.S. Food and Drug Administration (FDA) have not evaluated the statements made in this book. The products listed are not intended to diagnose, treat, cure, or prevent any disease.

Using any medication whether prescription, over the counter, or herbal in nature may have a marked effect on your health and each medicine may interact with others. Tell your health care provider about any complementary, supplemental, or alternative practices you use including dietary substances, herbals, or oils.

Federal regulations for dietary supplements are different from the regulations applied to prescription and over the counter drugs.

Dietary supplement manufacturers are not required to prove a product's safety and effectiveness.

Herbs and oils are sometimes marketed as dietary supplements. Herbs and oils do have a noticeable affect on the human body. The expected action of many herbs and oils is based on traditional use and observation. Laboratory studies have been conducted to confirm the expected affect of some traditionally used herbs and oils but others have not been well researched. Most dietary supplements, herbs, and oils have not been researched for use by pregnant women, nursing women, or children.

Each person's needs and correct dosage will vary depending on a variety of factors. You should discuss your specific needs and best dosage with our physician or qualified herbalist.

If you are thinking of using a dietary supplement for nutritional, supplement or other purpose, you should discuss your decision and alternatives with a physician or qualified herbalist.

I0446996

Introduction

Introduction

Normal, healthy skin is a beautiful sight, but many of us need a little help to keep our skin looking & feeling great.

Psoriasis is one of the most common skin diseases treated by dermatologists. Psoriasis is sometimes confused with eczema, another common skin disease. This confusion is caused mainly by the fact that the appearance of both diseases can be very similar. It is important to understand that the underlying cause of each disease is very different and to determine which one you have before starting any treatment program. You should consult with a dermatologist to obtain a diagnosis.

Once you have confirmed that psoriasis is the problem, there are lifestyle changes, natural topical preparations, and supplements that you can use to help reduce the number and severity of psoriasis flares that you experience.

There are multiple types of psoriasis but the most common is plaque psoriasis. Plaque psoriasis is most frequently found in adults. Plaque psoriasis causes areas of skin to become itchy and inflamed. Plaque psoriasis scales most commonly form on the back and lower body but can appear almost anywhere.

Psoriasis typically appears as reddish lesions with itchy, silvery scales that flake off and sometimes cause bleeding and scarring. The scales produced during a psoriasis outbreak are believed to be produced when the immune system sends signals to that speed up the growth cycle of skin cells.

Psoriasis can appear over many parts of the body including the back, chest, face, legs, and stomach among others. Different areas of your body will respond better to different treatments. You also want to use care when treating psoriasis flares because you do not want to cause other damage to the skin with the treatments. The recipes in this book include preparations that work better delicate skin like facial areas as well as preparations that work well on tougher body skin. You should always consider the sensitivity of your skin before using any preparation.

Before using topical and supplemental preparations to reduce the number and severity of psoriasis flares, you should consider some of the common triggers of psoriasis outbreaks. It may be possible to reduce your personal number of flares by simple lifestyle change.

Genetic predisposition is believed to play a large role in determining who gets psoriasis, however, not everyone who has the gene actually develops visible psoriasis symptoms. It is commonly believed that In addition to the genetic predisposition, a person has to be exposed to a trigger for psoriasis to become active. Each person may be sensitive to a different trigger that activates the disease and causes flares. These triggers are very individualized but some common triggers show up in the history of many psoriasis sufferers. Psoriasis is very specific to each individual so you should start by considering your lifestyle and potential flare triggers. Each person may have one or more triggers that need to be corrected before the psoriasis outbreaks can be minimized.

Increased stress or other psychological triggers may cause psoriasis flares. The exact mechanism that links stress to psoriasis is not clearly understood but there may be a relationship to the hormonal changes caused by stress.

If stress may be a trigger for your psoriasis, you should find a relaxation technique that helps to lower the hormonal changes related to stress and anxiety. While you cannot affect the hormonal changes that are a natural part of growing older, you can minimize the effect that stress and anxiety have on your life by learning a meditation or relaxation technique that works well for you.

Psoriasis outbreaks often appear on areas of the skin that have been injured. This injury can be a result of weather like sun or windburn, due to injury related to activity, or from another cause entirely. The key is to avoid common causes of injury to the skin, to protect your skin from the elements, and to treat any injury as soon as possible.

Some medications are believed to trigger a psoriasis flares. You should discuss any medication that you take with your dermatologist to see if there is a possible link between the medication and the appearance of new psoriasis scales. If there appears to be a link, your physician or a qualified herbalist may be able to assist you in finding alternative treatments to replace the medications.

Some people seem to find a link between their diet and their psoriasis outbreaks. This potential trigger has not been well documented but is an avenue worth exploring in your attempt to minimize the number and severity of your psoriasis flares. You should spend some time logging the items in your diet and see if you can locate a link between certain types of food products and psoriasis outbreaks. There is some controversy over whether diet really causes flares and additional research is constantly

being undertaken to confirm or rule out food as a cause. In the meantime, you can conduct your own personal research by logging intake and outbreaks to see if there is a personal link for you.

Once you have located the potential triggers of your psoriasis, you will have a better idea of how to treat and even prevent future flares.

The recipes in this book have been compiled to help treat the symptoms of psoriasis and to potentially minimize the number and severity of future outbreaks. These recipes have been created for the use of people who are close to me. You can try the recipes as they are written, or refer to the ingredient guide in the back of the recipe book to see if an alternative ingredient might work better for your particular situation. Remember, each person will have a slightly different situation including triggers, skin type, environment, and genetic history. You should experiment to find the perfect solution for you!

Natural care is about more than just using nature to solve a problem. Natural care is about CUSTOMIZING nature to solve your personal problem!

Soaps

The first step to beautiful, healthy skin is cleansing. You need to find the cleansing products that work best for your particular skin care needs. Before you can use any other product in your regimen the area you are treating must be clean. People sometimes overlook the importance of using the correct soap.

Consider that soap is the first item, and often the last, that you use each day. People often spend the rest of the day using products to counteract the effects of the soap they have chosen. Using the correct soap can either harm or enhance the rest of your products.

Some people prefer soft soap and that is my favorite method for cleaning my face. Other people prefer a harder soap, especially for body care.

Before deciding which soap recipe to try, you should understand the basics of skin and skin care. Many factors can affect the condition and appearance of skin. No soap or other product can replace simple daily care in your activities. Skin is the largest organ you have and perhaps the most important in that it protects every other part of you from environmental factors. Of course, skin is also very important because it is the first thing most people will notice about you.

The type of soap base and customization ingredients used in soap recipes is very specific to the individual and the problems that each individual might need to address. Soap can be a wonderful addition to both preventative and treatments for those who suffer from psoriasis.

You should select the soap that best meets your personal skin type, lifestyle, and needs and then customize the soap to include ingredients that have proven beneficial in the treatment and prevention of psoriasis.

This chapter outlines the creation of the most common types of soap that you can then customize to suit your needs. I have also included a few of my favorite soap customizations for you to use as a starting point. Remember to experiment – most of the ingredients in soap making are extremely cost effective and easy to locate. The more you experiment the more effective the product will be for your specific needs.

Do not be discouraged by the processes described since soap is a common item that has been successfully created by individuals for generations. To create exceptional soaps you just need to practice and perfect your skills. You will also need some dedicated equipment to create soap. You can easily find these items in specialty craft stores or often in an all-in-one retail chain. Some stores even carry kits that contain most of the key equipment in one package.

Cleansing is one of the best places that you can spend time experimenting and customizing the recipes to suit your needs. The better customized your cleansing regimen is to your particular skin type, lifestyle, and needs the better your appearance will be.

You may need to use different cleansers on different parts of your skin. Facial psoriasis tends to be a slightly different problem than the skin on the rest of your body and will need different treatments and preventatives.

Regardless of the recipes you choose to try it is always recommended that you test sample the products on a sensitive area such as your wrist to ensure that you do not have unexpected reactions before applying them to your skin. This is not a fail proof method of ensuring that the products are correct for you but it can often provide a warning of a negative reaction.

You should also look up each ingredient in the ingredient listing to determine potential side effects of using any natural ingredients. Natural products contain medicinal qualities just like prescription treatments and you need to ensure that each inclusion is safe and effective for your personal needs.

Basic Supplies

Thermometer –   Successful soap making depends heavily on temperature.

The base components like lye, borax, and fat must be heated to a particular temperature and then cooled to become soap.

A good method of ensuring that you reach the proper temperatures is to buy a decent candy thermometer for use in your soap making.

The thermometer should be used only for one particular type of soap and should be dedicated only to soap making. If you decide to experiment with soaps that have a variety of bases you will want to obtain a few thermometers since using the same thermometer for lye that you use for fat bases can throw off the results of your soap-making endeavor.

Thermometers can be found in most craft stores or in the cooking section of your grocery store. The thermometer you select does not need to be the most advanced or expensive model available. A simple, cost-effective thermometer will work just fine for these recipes.

Cooking Pot -   You will need a glass or steel pot for heating and mixing.

You should have a dedicated mixing container for your soap making endeavors. While most of the ingredients in soap are safe, you would not want to eat out of the same pan you just used for boiling lye. You also want to be careful not to transfer foods, spices, and other cooking matter into your soap. These can irritate or worsen the conditions you are trying to treat.

It is important not to use aluminum or iron pots and pans when creating soap. The metal in these pots can react with the ingredients of the soap. A basic steel or enamel-coated pot works best and is often the most cost-effective purchase. You can find these in most retail chain stores.

Wooden Utensils -   You will want to purchase a set of wooden utensils for soap making.

You should get a set of utensils that will be dedicated for use only with your product recipes. Again, these utensils should not be used for general cooking.

The type of utensils that have longer handles work well when making soap. You will need to stir deep into your cooking pots to ensure all the ingredients are well mixed and a longer handle makes it easier to stir and to prevent accidental contact between the ingredients and your hands.

Wooden utensils are heat resistant, will hold up better under some of the stronger ingredients you may choose to use, and will usually not cause an adverse reaction. You should not use metal utensils when making soap.

Gloves –   You will want to use a pair of kitchen gloves to protect your hands from the ingredients used in soap making.

You will use the final product of your soap making process on your skin, but the core ingredients can cause irritation or even burns before they are diluted into the recipe. Using a pair of kitchen gloves is the best practice during your soap making. These will protect your hands from inadvertent splashing and prevent problems that will then need to be treated using a different recipe.

Soap Molds -   You will need a mold or container to hold your completed soap during the hardening stage.

These recipes will often finish as a cake of soap. To achieve these perfectly formed cakes, you will need to use a mold. There are many molds available in specialty craft stores as well as at retail chain stores. Soap making has gained popularity in the last few years, making these products easier to find than ever before. You can find molds ranging from the very basic cake soap style to the more specialized styles that will suit your décor.

If you are using your soap yourself, you might not be as concerned with achieving the perfect appearance as you are with usefulness. You do not need to purchase specialized soap molds. Many items found in your house can be used as a mold.

You can use old baking pans such as muffin pans, cookie cutters, or bread pans as soap molds. You can even make your own mold out of old cardboard boxes. Almost any container that can withstand the heat of the liquid soap and will hold the liquid soap in place while it hardens will work as a mold.

Soap Making Dos!

When making soap, you must work in a well-ventilated area. Liquid and heated forms of some ingredients included in the soap making process can create fumes that may be harmful if inhaled.

Always wear gloves and other protective clothing when making soap since lye and other ingredients can burn or irritate the skin.

Always use COLD Distilled Water when mixing lye solutions.

Pour the lye mixture into the fat mixture not the other way around.

Keep solvents like vinegar nearby to neutralize the effect of the ingredients if they should touch the skin.

Remember that lye is a poison and should always be kept in a safe place.

Only create heated soap mixtures when you can be sure that you will not be distracted. Some of the ingredients and the heat processes involved in soap making can be dangerous. In addition, the recipes included in this chapter require a fine attention to detail to ensure success in your soap-making endeavor.

Beeswax Soap

Beeswax soap is becoming more popular for all types of treatments. The natural healing and antibacterial properties of beeswax make it a soap option with a wide range of uses. Beeswax also leaves a thin protective coating on the skin making it one of the better quality soaps for psoriasis treatment.

Creating this soap is sometimes a bit more expensive than the other forms since beeswax can be more costly. Check with your health food stores or a beekeeping compound in your area to find the best price on beeswax.

The following recipe will make approximately 1 bar of soap. You can enlarge it if you want to make a bigger batch.

Heat 1/3 cup of your favorite vegetable-based oil.

Review the optional ingredient list to determine which oil will provide the most beneficial effect for your needs.

Add 4 tsp. grated beeswax to the oils and heat until melted. The mixture will be approximately 90 degrees.

While your oils are heating, dissolve 2 tsp. lye in 1/3 cup cold distilled water.

Remember to wear protective gloves and clothing when working with lye since lye can burn your skin.

Store your unused lye granules in a safe place since lye is a poison.

Remove your oil mixture from the heat and allow it to allow cool slightly to approximately 70 degrees.

You will probably want to customize the soap mixture with the ingredients that best meet your particular needs. The recipes on the following pages will give you some starter ideas. The ingredient list included in this books glossary will give you a much more comprehensive idea of which additives will work best for you.

While I do use additives that can prove beneficial for certain conditions, I typically do not add color or fragrance to any product designed for damaged or sensitive skin because additives can cause the irritation to worsen. If you prefer something other than the natural color or scent, you can add your favorite colorant, essential oils or herbs to the mixture.

Slowly pour the lye solution into the oil mixture.

Stir the mixture gently but well to ensure that all of the ingredients are blended.

If the soap mixture does not thicken within 30 minutes or if there is a greasy layer on the top of the mixture it may be too warm.

Set the container in a pan of cool water.

Continue stirring, making sure to stir the sides and bottom of the pan to ensure an even mix.

The mixture will become thicker taking on the consistency of syrup.

If the soap mixture is too lumpy, it may be too cold. If this occurs, reverse the above process.

Sit the mixture in a pan of warm water stirring until the lumps dissolve. You may need to replace the warm water more than once until the mixture is heated to the correct temperature for effective blending.

Remember that everyone's skin reacts differently. You should test the products on a less sensitive area before using them. You should also remember that even natural products have side effects. The appendix gives the most common expected benefits and results of these ingredients. You should review these entries before trying any recipe.

Pour the thickened mixture into your molds, cover, and keep it in a warm place for at least 2 days. This helps to keep the mixture from separating.

Once the soap has set, remove the finished soap from the molds and cut it into bars.

Place the soap in a dry area until you are ready to use it.

Castile Soap

A nice soap base alternative to traditional bars is castile soap. To be castile soap the mixture must contain at least 40% olive oil. You can purchase ready-made castile soap and then customize the mixture to suit your needs or you may create castile soap at home.

This soap is especially mild and gentle making it a good selection for aging, damaged or irritated skin. Castile soap is a versatile soap, you can even use the same castile soap products to wash your hair as you use for the rest of your body. You should test castile soap on a smaller area before using it in treatments for acne since the oils may cause extra irritation in some people.

The following recipe will yield the liquid equivalent of 1 bar of soap. You can increase the recipe if you want to make a larger batch.

Heat 1/3 cup of olive oil to approximately 90 degrees Fahrenheit.

While the oil is heating, dissolve 2 tsp. lye granules in 1/3 cup cold water.

Remember to wear protective gloves and clothing when working with lye since lye can burn your skin. Store your unused lye granules in a safe place because lye is a poison.

Remove your oil mixture from the heat and allow it to cool slightly to approximately 70 degrees.

You will probably want to customize the soap mixture with the ingredients that best meet your particular needs. The recipes on the following pages will give you some starter ideas. The ingredient list included in this books glossary will give you a much more comprehensive idea of which additives will work best for you.

While I do use additives that can prove beneficial for certain conditions, I typically do not add color or fragrance to any product designed for damaged or sensitive skin because additives can cause the irritation to worsen. If you prefer something other than the natural color or scent, you can add your favorite colorant, essential oils or herbs to the mixture.

Slowly pour the lye solution into the oil mixture.

Stir the mixture gently but well to ensure that all of the ingredients are well blended.

Allow the mixture to cool before placing it in a dispenser jar. If you want to convert liquid castile soap to a bar product, you will add a thickening agent and emulsifier and pour the finished mixture into molds as you would with any bar soap.

Remember that everyone's skin reacts differently. You should test the products on a less sensitive area before using them. You should also remember that even natural products have side effects. The appendix gives the most common expected benefits and results of these ingredients. You should review these entries before trying any recipe.

Coconut Oil Soap

Coconut oil is an excellent skin protectant and is one of the nicest natural foaming products that you can find to use in the soap making process

The following recipe will yield approximately 1 bar of soap. You can increase the recipe if you want a bigger batch.

Heat 3 teaspoons of coconut oil and ¼-cup vegetable-based oil on low heat to approximately 75 degrees Fahrenheit.

While the mixture is heating, dissolve 2 tsp. lye granules in 1/3 cup cold water.

Remember to wear protective gloves and clothing when working with lye since lye can burn your skin.

Store your unused lye granules in a safe place because lye is a poison.

Remove your oil mixture from the heat and allow it to cool slightly to approximately 70 degrees.

You will probably want to customize the soap mixture with the ingredients that best meet your particular needs. The recipes on the following pages will give you some starter ideas. The ingredient list included in this books glossary will give you a much more comprehensive idea of which additives will work best for you.

While I do use additives that can prove beneficial for certain conditions, I typically do not add color or fragrance to any product designed for damaged or sensitive skin because additives can cause the irritation to worsen. If you prefer something other than the natural color or scent, you can add your favorite colorant, essential oils or herbs to the mixture.

Slowly pour the lye solution into the oil mixture. Stir until the ingredients are well blended

If the soap mixture does not thicken within 30 minutes or there is a greasy layer on the top of the mixture it may be too warm.

Set the container in a pan of cool water. Stir the mixture, making certain that you stir the sides and bottom of the pan to ensure an even mix.

The mixture will become thicker taking on the consistency of syrup.

If the soap is lumpy, your mixture may be too cold. If this occurs, reverse the above process.

Sit the mixture in a pan of warm water stirring until the lumps dissolve. Depending on the consistency you may need to replace your warm water more than once until the mixture is heated to the correct temperature for effective blending.

Pour the thickened mixture into your molds, cover, and keep the mixture in a warm place for at least 2 days. This helps keep the soap from separating.

Remember that everyone's skin reacts differently. You should test the products on a less sensitive area before using them. You should also remember that even natural products have side effects. The appendix gives the most common expected benefits and results of these ingredients. You should review these entries before trying any recipe.

Tallow Based Soaps

Tallow has been used for generations in soap making and is considered one of the most common homemade soap products. Tallow soaps are made using the fat by-product trimmed from meat. You can collect clean fat as you cook. Simply trim off clean beef or pork fat before you cook your meat and save it, preferably in the freezer, until you are ready to make soap. Your local butcher or meat department will often provide you with free fat that is left when they trim their products.

One bar of soap will need approximately 1 cup of clean fat. You can increase the recipe if you want to create a bigger batch.

Place the fat in your soap-making pan and heat it until it is melted to an oil form.

Allow your mixture to cool to approximately 115 degrees Fahrenheit.

Add 1 tsp. of borax powder for each cup of melted fat. You do not have to add borax but it does give a better appearance and lather to your soap. If you add the borax, stir the powder into your tallow mixture until well blended.

You will probably want to customize the soap mixture with the ingredients that best meet your particular needs. The recipes on the following pages will give you some starter ideas. The ingredient list included in this books glossary will give you a much more comprehensive idea of which additives will work best for you.

While I do use additives that can prove beneficial for certain conditions, I typically do not add color or fragrance to any product designed for damaged or sensitive skin because additives can cause the irritation to worsen. If you prefer something other than the natural color or scent, you can add your favorite colorant, essential oils or herbs to the mixture.

While your tallow mixture is cooling to the desired temperature, you will need to create the lye solution. Again, remember to wear protective gloves and clothing when using lye because it can burn the skin.

Lye is a poison and unused amounts should be stored in a safe place.

Dissolve the lye granules in cool water.

You will use approximately 3 teaspoons of lye to ½-cup water for each bar of soap being created.

Once the lye granules are dissolved, you will slowly pour the lye mixture into the fat mixture.

Pour it in a slow steady stream while stirring the mixture.

You should not have the heat on the mixture at this time.

Stir the ingredients until thick syrup is formed. This should take approximately 10-20 minutes.

If the soap is not becoming thick after 30 minutes or has a greasy layer floating on the top, the mixture may be too warm.

Set the container in a pan of cool water.

Continue stirring, making sure to stir the sides and bottom of the pan to ensure an even mix.

If the soap is too lumpy, your mixture may be too cold.

If this occurs, reverse the above process.

Sit the mixture in a pan of warm water stirring until the lumps dissolve.

Depending on the consistency of the mixture, you may need to replace your warm Distilled Water more than once until the soap is heated to the correct temperature.

Pour the thickened mixture into your molds, cover, and keep the mixture in a warm place for at least 2 days. This helps to keep the mixture from separating.

Once the soap has set, remove it from the molds and place it a dry area to age. Aging soap ensures a better quality final soap product. You should allow your tallow soap to age at least 2-3 weeks prior to use.

At times, you will find that your soap is lumpy or has separated during the aging process. If this occurs, do not throw out the failed soap.

Cut the flawed cakes of soap into small pieces. You can use an ordinary kitchen grater to cut the soap into smaller pieces.

Return the pieces to your soap-making pan and add approximately 1 cup of Distilled Water for each cake of ground soap.

Dissolve the soap in the water over low heat. Stir the mixture occasionally to help distribute the heat.

When the lumps have disappeared and the mixture has formed a syrup, pour the soap into your favorite molds and follow the process for storage outlined earlier.

This will often cure the problem and provide you with a successful soap.

Remember that everyone's skin reacts differently. You should test the products on a less sensitive area before using them. You should also remember that even natural products have side effects. The appendix gives the most common expected benefits and results of these ingredients. You should review these entries before trying any recipe.

Glycerin Soap

One of the most common homemade cake soaps is a glycerin-based soap.

Glycerin is found naturally in many plants and is actually a by-product of the tallow soap making process. When making a fat and lye soap there is often a clear, thick liquid that floats on the top of the mixture. This is glycerin.

Glycerin soap is simply a basic soap that has extra glycerin added to the mixture. This soap is excellent for all skin types because it tends to be very mild. Glycerin is also natural humectant that draws and retains moisture in your skin.

The following recipe will make approximately 1 bar of soap. You can increase the recipe if you want to make a bigger batch.

Heat 1/3 cup of your favorite vegetable-based oil to approximately 90 degrees. Review the oil ingredient list to determine which oil will provide the most beneficial effect for your needs.

Add 1 tsp. of borax powder for each bar of soap you are making. You do not need to add the borax powder but it will make a nicer final product. If you choose to add the borax powder to your soap, stir the oils and borax until they are well blended.

While your oils are heating, dissolve 2 tsp. lye in 1/3 cup cold water.

Remember to wear protective gloves and clothing when working with lye since it can burn your skin.

Store your unused lye granules in a safe place because lye is a poison.

Remove your oil mixture from the heat and allow it to cool to approximately 70 degrees.

You will probably want to customize the soap mixture with the ingredients that best meet your particular needs. The recipes on the following pages will give you some starter ideas. The ingredient list included in this books glossary will give you a much more comprehensive idea of which additives will work best for you.

While I do use additives that can prove beneficial for certain conditions, I typically do not add color or fragrance to any product designed for damaged or sensitive skin because additives can cause the irritation to worsen. If you prefer something other than the natural color or scent, you can add your favorite colorant, essential oils or herbs to the mixture.

Slowly pour the lye solution into the oil mixture.

Stir the mixture gently but mix well to ensure all of the ingredients are well blended.

When the ingredients are well blended, add 3 tsp. glycerin.

Continue stirring the mixture until the ingredients are well blended.

The mixture will take on the consistency of syrup.

If the soap mixture does not thicken within 30 minutes or if there is a greasy layer on the top of the mixture, it may be too warm.

Set the container in a pan of cool water.

Continue stirring, making sure to stir the sides and bottom of the pan to ensure an even mix.

If the soap mixture is too lumpy, your mixture may be too cold. If this occurs, reverse the above process.

Sit the mixture in a pan of warm water stirring until the lumps dissolve.

Depending on the consistency, you may need to replace your warm water more than once until the lumps dissolve.

Pour the thickened mixture into your molds, cover, and keep it in a warm place for at least 2 days. This helps to keep the mixture from separating.

Remember that everyone's skin reacts differently. You should test the products on a less sensitive area before using them. You should also remember that even natural products have side effects. The appendix gives the most common expected benefits and results of these ingredients. You should review these entries before trying any recipe.

Soap Variations

The soap recipes on the following pages provide some customizations that you can use with the soap base recipes. You can create your own soap using the recipes on the previous pages, purchase melt-and-pour soap from a natural product supplier, or buy mass-market soap to use as a base. You will then customize these bases with ingredients that suit your particular skin care needs.

The variations on these pages are some of my favorite soap customizations. The ingredient mixes will work well with any of the core soap bases described earlier. At times, there is a soap base that works exceptionally well for a particular customization. These are noted in the recipe as a suggestion.

Remember that everyone's skin reacts differently. You should test the products on a less sensitive area before using them. You should also remember that even natural products have side effects. The appendix gives the most common expected benefits and results of these ingredients. You should review these entries before trying any recipe.

Do not be afraid to replace an ingredient in the recipes if you feel there is a better alternative for your needs. Creating your own natural products is all about experimentation and customization. You should strive to use the ingredients that meet your particular needs in every recipe.

Soothing Oatmeal Soap

Perhaps my favorite soap modification is to add oatmeal to my soap base giving me a cleansing but soothing soap product. Oatmeal is gentle, soothing, and cleansing all at the same time. Oatmeal adds an exfoliating effect to the soap mixture while providing a soft, moist feel to the skin. Liquid based oatmeal soap is very versatile so a Castile base is an excellent choice. I also love adding these ingredients to my coconut oil soap. This is a nice exfoliating and moisturizing option for reducing the appearance of psoriasis scales while infusing moisture into dry damaged skin. The safflower oil is believed to discourage cell proliferation making it a perfect choice for psoriasis recipes.

1 tsp.	Soapwort Powder – You can use Borax if desired
1/3 cup	Safflower Oil
1 tsp.	Coconut Oil

Heat the soapwort and oil mixture to approximately 90 degrees in your soap-making pan, in the microwave, or using a double broiler. Remove the mixture from the heat and set it aside to cool to about 70 degrees.

Soapwort is not a necessary ingredient for this recipe but it can improve the appearance and performance of your soap.

Mix well and add

3 tsp.	Glycerin
¼ cup	Oatmeal - Ground
	Fragrance, Color, Emulsifier & Thickener as desired

While I do add herbs & oils that contain beneficial compounds, I typically do not add color or fragrance to any product designed for damaged skin because additives can cause the irritation to worsen. If you prefer something other than the natural color or scent, you can add your favorite colorant, essential oils or herbs to the mixture.

Pour the blended ingredients into your favorite soap base.

You may need to heat the mixture a second time before blending it with your soap base.

Continue stirring the mixture until the ingredients are well blended.

The mixture will become thicker as you stir. Pour the finished product into the soap molds of your choice and allow it to harden and age as directed by the soap base instructions.

Remember that everyone's skin reacts differently. You should test the products on a less sensitive area before using them. You should also remember that even natural products have side effects. The appendix gives the most common expected benefits and results of these ingredients. You should review these entries before trying any recipe.

Psoriasis Reversing Bar

This fantastic moisturizing soap also acts to counter the redness, itchiness, and scale formation of a psoriasis outbreak. The neem & safflower oil blend is one of the best options I have found for reducing the severity of an active outbreak while reducing the duration by slowing the growth of new scales. This recipe works best with a glycerin or coconut oil base.

1/3 cup	Safflower Oil
2 tbsp.	Neem Oil
1 tsp.	Glycerin

Heat the oils & glycerin to approximately 90 degrees in your soap-making pan, in the microwave, or using a double broiler.

Remove your oil mixture from the heat and allow it to cool to approximately 70 degrees.

3 tbsp.	Powdered Seaweed

Add the powdered seaweed to the oils and stir the mixture until the ingredients are well blended.

While I do add herbs & oils that contain beneficial compounds, I typically do not add color or fragrance to any product designed for damaged skin because additives can cause the irritation to worsen. If you prefer something other than the natural color or scent, you can add your favorite colorant, essential oils or herbs to the mixture.

Pour the blended ingredients into your favorite soap base.

You may need to heat the mixture a second time before blending it with your soap base.

Continue stirring the mixture until the ingredients are well blended.

The mixture will become thicker as you stir. Pour the finished product into the soap molds of your choice and allow it to harden and age as directed by the soap base instructions.

Remember that everyone's skin reacts differently. You should test the products on a less sensitive area before using them. You should also remember that even natural products have side effects. The appendix gives the most common expected benefits and results of these ingredients. You should review these entries before trying any recipe.

Double I Bars

We call these the Double I bars since they act to reduce both inflammation and itchiness associated with psoriasis. These bars have a lovely scent and are one of our favorite choices for morning cleansing.

3 tbsp.   Safflower Oil

3 tbsp.   Baobab Oil

3 tbsp.   Golden Seal Oil

3 tbsp.   Lavender Oil

1 tbsp.   Honey

2 tbsp.   Aloe Vera Gel

Create your soap base according to the instructions for the soap that you want t o use for this recipe. I prefer glycerin soap as a base for this recipe.

Cool the soap base to approximately 70 degrees and add the modification ingredients. Stir until the ingredients are well blended in your soap base.

While I do add herbs & oils that contain beneficial compounds, I typically do not add color or fragrance to any product designed for damaged skin because additives can cause the irritation to worsen. If you prefer something other than the natural color or scent, you can add your favorite colorant, essential oils or herbs to the mixture.

Pour the blended ingredients into your favorite soap base.

Continue stirring the mixture until the ingredients are well blended.

The mixture will become thicker as you stir. Pour the finished product into the soap molds of your choice and allow it to harden and age as directed by the soap base instructions.

Remember that everyone's skin reacts differently. You should test the products on a less sensitive area before using them. You should also remember that even natural products have side effects. The appendix gives the most common expected benefits and results of these ingredients. You should review these entries before trying any recipe.

Healing Apple Soap

An excellent soap choice for irritated skin is apple juice based soap. This is great when you have itchy, irritated skin and works wonders for treating skin overstressed by environmental factors. The juice helps to attract moisture, the beeswax protects from irritants, and the honey locust helps to speed healing of areas where the scales have been scraped from the skin.

4 tsp.   Grated Beeswax

Heat the beeswax to approximately 90 degrees until it has formed a loose liquid.

Remove your oil mixture from the heat and allow it to cool to approximately 70 degrees. Add

2 tbsp.   Apple Juice

1 tsp.   Liquid Chlorophyll

1 tsp.   Honey Locust Thorn Juice

The mixture will have a delicate apple scent and a lovely green color. If you desire a different color or fragrance, you may add food coloring or the desired essential oils to the mixture.

While I do add herbs & oils that contain beneficial compounds, I typically do not add color or fragrance to any product designed for damaged skin because additives can cause the irritation to worsen.

The mixture will become thicker as you stir. Pour the finished product into the soap molds of your choice and allow it to harden and age as directed by the soap base instructions.

Remember that everyone's skin reacts differently. You should test the products on a less sensitive area before using them. You should also remember that even natural products have side effects. The appendix gives the most common expected benefits and results of these ingredients. You should review these entries before trying any recipe.

Healing & Hydrating Bars

This soap is an excellent choice when you want to hydrate skin while stimulating healing. The soap leaves the skin feeling clean & refreshed while acting to reduce inflammation and speed the healing of psoriasis scales. You will be amazed at how moist and clear you skin looks after using this soap.

1 cup	Distilled Water
½ tsp.	Powdered Sarsaparilla
½ tsp.	Powdered Mallow Root

Add the mallow root & sarsaparilla to the water and heat the mixture to a light boil. Allow the mixture to boil until approximately ½ of the water has boiled off. This will leave ½ cup of very dark tea. Strain the mallow root & sarsaparilla from the water and discard the plant materials. The ½ cup of fluid that remains will act as your soap base.

1 tsp.	Soapwort
1 tsp.	Costus Oil
2 tsp.	Grated Beeswax

Melt the beeswax until it reaches around 90 degrees Fahrenheit and has a liquid appearance. Remove the beeswax from the heat and add the soapwort powder & oil to the base. Soapwort is not a necessary ingredient for this recipe but it can improve the appearance and performance of your soap.

Blend the mallow root & sarsaparilla liquid into the beeswax base.

2 tsp.	Lye Granules
1/3 cup	Cold Water

In a separate pan, dissolve the lye granules in cold water. Slowly pour the lye blend into the beeswax mixture. Stir the liquid until the ingredients are well blended.

If you desire a specific color or fragrance for your soap, you may add your favorite food coloring or essential oils.

While I do add herbs & oils that contain beneficial compounds, I typically do not add color or fragrance to any product designed for damaged skin because additives can cause the irritation to worsen.

Pour the solution of your choice into the base. You can simply increase the amount of beeswax to instead of adding a soap base. This will help the mixture to solidify.

Continue stirring the mixture until well blended. The mixture will become thicker taking on the consistency of syrup.

Pour the finished product into the soap molds of your choice and allow it to harden and age as directed by the soap base instructions.

Remember that everyone's skin reacts differently. You should test the products on a less sensitive area before using them. You should also remember that even natural products have side effects. The appendix gives the most common expected benefits and results of these ingredients. You should review these entries before trying any recipe.

Scar Reduction Bars

One of the hardest issues to remedy is the darkening that sometimes remains after a psoriasis outbreak. This pigmentation can take the form or spotting in a localized spot or a darker cast to an entire area. This beeswax soap modification is wonderful for hydrating and soothing damaged skin while helping to lighten the natural darkening that can occur because of psoriasis.

1/4 cup	Safflower Oil
2 tbsp.	Grated Beeswax
1 tbsp.	Honey

Heat the mixture for approximately 25 seconds on medium heat in the microwave or to approximately 90 degrees in a double broiler. The melted ingredients will take on a syrupy consistency.

Remove your oil mixture from the heat and allow it to cool to approximately 70 degrees. Add

2 tbsp.	Bitter Damson - Powdered
½ tsp.	Andiroba Oil
½ tsp.	Kukui Nut Oil

While I do add herbs & oils that contain beneficial compounds, I typically do not add color or fragrance to any product designed for damaged skin because additives can cause the irritation to worsen. If you prefer something other than the natural color or scent, you can add your favorite colorant, essential oils or herbs to the mixture.

Pour the soap solution of your choice into the oil mixture and blend well.

The mixture will become thicker as you stir. Pour the finished product into the soap molds of your choice and allow it to harden and age as directed by the soap base instructions.

Remember that everyone's skin reacts differently. You should test the products on a less sensitive area before using them. You should also remember that even natural products have side effects. The appendix gives the most common expected benefits and results of these ingredients. You should review these entries before trying any recipe.

Skin Brightening Bars

Psoriasis scales can sometimes leave darkened areas or pigmentation scars behind after they have healed. Reducing the appearance of dark pigmentation is an important step to making sure that your skin looks wonderful after a psoriasis flare. Another important step is to brighten & tone the skin. These bars help to fade pigmentation scars and brighten the skin while adding a nice toned, hydrated look.

1/4 cup   Coconut Oil

2 tbsp.   Grated Beeswax

1 tbsp.   Safflower Seed Oil

Heat the mixture for approximately 25 seconds on medium heat in the microwave or to approximately 90 degrees in a double broiler. The melted ingredients will take on a syrupy consistency.

Remove your oil mixture from the heat and allow it to cool to approximately 70 degrees.   Add

2 tbsp.   Powdered Fumitory

½ tsp.   Geranium Oil

While I do add herbs & oils that contain beneficial compounds, I typically do not add color or fragrance to any product designed for damaged skin because additives can cause the irritation to worsen. If you prefer something other than the natural color or scent, you can add your favorite colorant, essential oils or herbs to the mixture.

Pour the soap solution of your choice into the oil mixture and blend well.

The mixture will become thicker as you stir. Pour the finished product into the soap molds of your choice and allow it to harden and age as directed by the soap base instructions.

Remember that everyone's skin reacts differently. You should test the products on a less sensitive area before using them. You should also remember that even natural products have side effects. The appendix gives the most common expected benefits and results of these ingredients. You should review these entries before trying any recipe.

Toning Bars

This is an amazing skin-toning recipe that helps to infuse moisture and reduce the appearance of psoriasis while gently toning and tightening the skin.

1/4 cup	Almond Oil
2 tbsp.	Grated Beeswax
1 tbsp.	Honey

Heat the mixture for approximately 25 seconds on medium heat in the microwave or to approximately 90 degrees in a double broiler. The melted ingredients will take on a syrupy consistency.

Remove your oil mixture from the heat and allow it to cool to approximately 70 degrees.   Add

2 tbsp.	Powdered Bittersweet Twigs
2 tsp.	Club Moss Spore Powder
1 tsp.	Borax Powder
2 tsp.	Fennel Oil

Stir the mixture until the ingredients are well blended.

While I do add herbs & oils that contain beneficial compounds, I typically do not add color or fragrance to any product designed for damaged skin because additives can cause the irritation to worsen. If you prefer something other than the natural color or scent, you can add your favorite colorant, essential oils or herbs to the mixture.

Pour the soap solution of your choice into the oil mixture and blend well.

The mixture will become thicker as you stir. Pour the finished product into the soap molds of your choice and allow it to harden and age as directed by the soap base instructions.

Remember that everyone's skin reacts differently. You should test the products on a less sensitive area before using them. You should also remember that even natural products have side effects. The appendix gives the most common expected benefits and results of these ingredients. You should review these entries before trying any recipe.

Collagen Building Bars

Collagen building may not be the perfect solution for your particular needs depending on the type and causes of your psoriasis outbreaks. If your psoriasis results in pitting and saggy skin or if you have aging skin, building collagen may be a critical element to helping your skin to look and feel wonderful between psoriasis flares. This bar recipe contains light collagen stimulating properties that help to reduce the appearance of pitting, a type of post-outbreak scarring.

1/4 cup	Sunflower Oil
2 tbsp.	Grated Beeswax
2 tbsp.	Grape Seed Oil

Heat the mixture for approximately 25 seconds on medium heat in the microwave or to approximately 90 degrees in a double broiler. The melted ingredients will take on a syrupy consistency.

Remove your oil mixture from the heat and allow it to cool to approximately 70 degrees. Add

2 tbsp.	Gotu Kola
½ tsp.	Myrrh Oil
½ tsp.	Immortelle

While I do add herbs & oils that contain beneficial compounds, I typically do not add color or fragrance to any product designed for damaged skin because additives can cause the irritation to worsen. If you prefer something other than the natural color or scent, you can add your favorite colorant, essential oils or herbs to the mixture.

Pour the soap solution of your choice into the oil mixture and blend well.

The mixture will become thicker as you stir. Pour the finished product into the soap molds of your choice and allow it to harden and age as directed by the soap base instructions.

Remember that everyone's skin reacts differently. You should test the products on a less sensitive area before using them. You should also remember that even natural products have side effects. The appendix gives the most common expected benefits and results of these ingredients. You should review these entries before trying any recipe.

Silkening Bars

Sometimes, we need to concentrate on pampering our skin, not just reducing the appearance of psoriasis. This soap not only helps to tighten the skin, it adds a lovely, supple feeling. It also helps to discourage the formation of new scales acting as a preventative against future psoriasis flares. I love to use these bars whenever my skin is healthy overall and I can spend some time pampering.

1/4 cup	Safflower Oil
4 tsp.	Grated Beeswax

Heat the mixture for approximately 25 seconds on medium heat in the microwave or to approximately 90 degrees in a double broiler. The melted ingredients will take on a syrupy consistency.

Remove your oil mixture from the heat and allow it to cool to approximately 70 degrees. Add

2 tbsp.	Evening Primrose Oil
2 tbsp.	Glycerin
3 tbsp.	Cajuput Oils

Stir the mixture until all of the ingredients are well blended.

While I do add herbs & oils that contain beneficial compounds, I typically do not add color or fragrance to any product designed for damaged skin because additives can cause the irritation to worsen. If you prefer something other than the natural color or scent, you can add your favorite colorant, essential oils or herbs to the mixture.

Pour the soap solution of your choice into the oil mixture and blend well.

The mixture will become thicker as you stir. Pour the finished product into the soap molds of your choice and allow it to harden and age as directed by the soap base instructions.

Remember that everyone's skin reacts differently. You should test the products on a less sensitive area before using them. You should also remember that even natural products have side effects. The appendix gives the most common expected benefits and results of these ingredients. You should review these entries before trying any recipe.

Bedtime Bars

This is a favorite of mine at night before bed. The natural aroma of lavender and chamomile provide a relaxing benefit minimizing stress. This is especially important if your psoriasis outbreaks are linked to stress. The soap itself softens and hydrates the skin, reduces scales and speeds healing of damaged skin. I typically follow this treatment with a hydrating moisturizer and wake with beautiful, moisturized skin.

1 tsp.	Chamomile Leaves
1 tsp.	Speedwell
1/4 cup	Water

Heat the Distilled Water to the boiling point and pour it over the leaves. Do not immerse the leaves in boiling Distilled Water since this might minimize the beneficial compounds contained in the plant parts. Allow the leaves and Distilled Water to soak overnight. The mixture should form a very strong tea. You can stain the plant parts from the mixture or leave them in to give added power to the finished soap.

3 tbsp.	Grated Beeswax

Heat the beeswax for approximately 25 seconds on medium heat in the microwave or to approximately 90 degrees in a double broiler. The melted ingredients will take on a syrupy consistency. Remove mixture from the heat and allow it to cool to approximately 70 degrees.

1 tsp. Borax Powder

Dissolve the borax powder in the wax base. Borax in not a necessary ingredient for this recipe but it can improve the appearance and performance of your soap.

When the mixture is well blended, add the remaining ingredients.

1 tbsp.	Coconut Oil
3 tbsp .	Safflower Oil
3 tsp.	Lavender Oil
1 tsp.	Horse Chestnut Oil
3 tsp.	Glycerin

¼ cup   Wheat Germ

While I do add herbs & oils that contain beneficial compounds, I typically do not add color or fragrance to any product designed for damaged skin because additives can cause the irritation to worsen. If you prefer something other than the natural color or scent, you can add your favorite colorant, essential oils or herbs to the mixture.

Pour the soap solution of your choice into the oil mixture and blend well.

The mixture will become thicker as you stir. Pour the finished product into the soap molds of your choice and allow it to harden and age as directed by the soap base instructions.

Remember that everyone's skin reacts differently. You should test the products on a less sensitive area before using them. You should also remember that even natural products have side effects. The appendix gives the most common expected benefits and results of these ingredients. You should review these entries before trying any recipe.

Soft Soaps & Cleansers

Every inch of your skin is important and deserves to be treated with care but certain areas require specialized attention. Soft soaps and cleansers are a preferred choice for some people, especially when treating facial skin or psoriasis scales. Soft cleansers help to remove the dirt, oils, flaky skin, and other issues that worsen the appearance, discomfort, and duration of a psoriasis flare.

Cleansing is one of the best places that you can spend time experimenting and customizing the recipes to suit your needs. The better customized your cleansing regimen is to your particular skin type, lifestyle, and needs the better your overall appearance will be.

You may need to use different cleansers on different parts of your skin. The face & neck area tends to need different treatments and preventatives than other skin like elbows & knees. You should consider the goal of the treatment, sensitivity of the areas being treated, and personal application preferences before selecting recipes to try.

Regardless of the recipes you choose to try it is always recommended that you test sample the products on a sensitive area such as your wrist to ensure that you do not have unexpected reactions before applying them to your skin. This is not a fail proof method of ensuring that the products are correct for you but it can often provide a warning of a negative reaction.

You should also look up each ingredient in the ingredient listing to determine potential side effects of using any natural product. Natural products contain medicinal qualities and you need to ensure that each inclusion is safe and effective for your personal needs.

Gentle Foaming Scrub

Foaming facial washes are one of my favorite types of cleansers. The foaming action helps to clean the skin and makes application a breeze. This is a favorite cleaner of mine since it is gentle enough for use on almost any skin. The ingredients help to tighten my skin, infuse moisture, and reduce the severity & duration of psoriasis flare up.

3 tbsp.	Coconut Oil
1 tbsp.	Safflower Oil
1 tbsp.	Neem Oil
1 tsp.	Fennel Oil
	Emulsifier & Thickener as desired

Gently stir the oils until they are well blended. Do not whip this recipe since the coconut oil will foam. If the coconut oil is too solid for blending, you can warm it between the palms of your hand to soften it.

This recipe has a delicate, sweet smell but if you desire a specific color or fragrance, you may add your favorite colorant or essential oils or herbs to the mixture.

While I do add herbs & oils that contain beneficial compounds, I typically do not add color or fragrance to any product designed for damaged skin because additives can cause the irritation to worsen.

Spoon mixture into a clean container and seal it tightly.

To use, place a small amount in the palm of your hand, mix with water, and scrub your face with a gentle upward motion. This is a soap mixture so always rinse your skin thoroughly when done washing.

Remember that everyone's skin reacts differently. You should test the products on a less sensitive area before using them. You should also remember that even natural products have side effects. The appendix gives the most common expected benefits and results of these ingredients. You should review these entries before trying any recipe.

Basic Daily Cleanser

This recipe is a nice, gentle cleanser that can be used on a daily basis to help combat future psoriasis flares and speed healing of current flares while helping to support the rest of your skin.

1 tbsp.	Birch Bark Powder
3 tbsp.	Witch Hazel
½ cup	Aloe Vera Gel
1 tbsp.	Gotu Kola Oil Emulsifier & Thickener as desired

Mix the ingredients in a blender or food processor until they are well blended.

While I do add herbs & oils that contain beneficial compounds, I typically do not add color or fragrance to any product designed for damaged skin because additives can cause the irritation to worsen. If you prefer something other than the natural color or scent, you can add your favorite colorant, essential oils or herbs to the mixture.

Pour the finished mixture into clean container and seal tightly.

To use, pour small amount in the palm of your hand or apply it with a gentle upward motion. Allow the mixture to sit on your skin for 30-60 seconds before rinsing. This is also an excellent cleanser to add to your favorite scrubbing sacks. This is a soap mixture so always rinse your skin thoroughly when done washing.

Remember that everyone's skin reacts differently. You should test the products on a less sensitive area before using them. You should also remember that even natural products have side effects. The appendix gives the most common expected benefits and results of these ingredients. You should review these entries before trying any recipe.

Daily Cleanser with Toning Agents

This recipe visibly reduces the appearance of pores while helping to combat the severity of a psoriasis outbreak. This cleanser provides a balm that helps heal damaged skin while giving a light toning action. I modify the recipe by adding ingredients from the alternate ingredient list throughout the year to get the most beneficial results for each season. You can use this cleanser alone or add additional ingredients from the list to ensure the best results for your skin type.

2 tbsp.	Oak Gall Extract
3 tsp.	Honey
¼ cup	Rosewater
1 tsp .	Borax Powder
1 tbsp.	Fennel Oil
	Emulsifier & Thickener as desired

Gently stir the ingredients until they are well blended.

While I do add herbs & oils that contain beneficial compounds, I typically do not add color or fragrance to any product designed for damaged skin because additives can cause the irritation to worsen. If you prefer something other than the natural color or scent, you can add your favorite colorant, essential oils or herbs to the mixture.

Store the mixture in a tightly sealed container. To use, massage a small amount into your skin using an upward motion. Let the mixture sit on the skin for 30 – 60 seconds before rinsing. This is a soap mixture so always rinse your skin thoroughly when done washing.

Remember that everyone's skin reacts differently. You should test the products on a less sensitive area before using them. You should also remember that even natural products have side effects. The appendix gives the most common expected benefits and results of these ingredients. You should review these entries before trying any recipe.

Daily Moisture Infusing Cleanser

This light cleanser combines moisture-infusing ingredients with a very gentle cleansing action. It makes a good selection for preventative daily cleansing helping to minimize the likelihood of new scale development while infusing moisture that will help to heal existing flakiness.

½ cup	Castile Soap
1/8 cup	Rose Hip Oil
1 tbsp.	Powdered Moneywort
1 tbsp.	Grape Seed Oil

Mix all of the ingredients until they are well blended.

While I do add herbs & oils that contain beneficial compounds, I typically do not add color or fragrance to any product designed for damaged skin because additives can cause the irritation to worsen. If you prefer something other than the natural color or scent, you can add your favorite colorant, essential oils or herbs to the mixture.

Pour the finished mixture into your favorite applicator bottle. This is a soap mixture so always rinse your skin thoroughly when done washing.

Castile soap can be made at home following the basic recipe in the soap making section.

Remember that everyone's skin reacts differently. You should test the products on a less sensitive area before using them. You should also remember that even natural products have side effects. The appendix gives the most common expected benefits and results of these ingredients. You should review these entries before trying any recipe.

Soothing Wash

This is a fantastic nighttime cleanser. Lavender gives a soothing effect that helps to combat psoriasis flares stimulated by stress while the other ingredients help to tighten, tone, and heal the skin. I also use it as a bath additive when I need a relaxing bath to help prepare for bed or a full body cleanser. Those who suffer from psoriasis flares related to stress might find this a good morning and evening cleansing choice.

¼ tsp	Tincture of Benzoin
1 tbsp	Distilled Water
3 tbsp	Witch Hazel
3-4 drops	Lavender Oil
1 tsp	Glycerin
3 tbsp	Aloe Vera Gel

Gently combine all of the ingredients until they well blended.

While I do add herbs & oils that contain beneficial compounds, I typically do not add color or fragrance to any product designed for damaged skin because additives can cause the irritation to worsen. If you prefer something other than the natural color or scent, you can add your favorite colorant, essential oils or herbs to the mixture.

Store the mixture in a tightly sealed container.

To use, massage a small amount into your skin using an upward motion. Let the mixture sit on the skin for 30 – 60 seconds before rinsing. This is a soap mixture so always rinse your skin thoroughly when done washing.

Remember that everyone's skin reacts differently. You should test the products on a less sensitive area before using them. You should also remember that even natural products have side effects. The appendix gives the most common expected benefits and results of these ingredients. You should review these entries before trying any recipe.

Collagen Building Balm

I like to use a collagen building soap on every part of my body. Everything from deep scarring after treating a severe psoriasis outbreak to skin sagging & wrinkling relates to the lack of collagen in the skin. This nice foaming cleanser blends some of my favorite collagen building & skin regenerating ingredients into a healing cleansing agent.

¼ cup   Aloe Vera Gel

1 tbsp.   Vitamin E Oil

2 tbsp.   Borax Powder

2 tbsp.   Myrrh Oil

1 tbsp.   Safflower Oil

¼ cup   Witch Hazel

  Dissolve borax powder in the witch hazel base. Add the remaining ingredients and blend well.

While I do add herbs & oils that contain beneficial compounds, I typically do not add color or fragrance to any product designed for damaged skin because additives can cause the irritation to worsen. If you prefer something other than the natural color or scent, you can add your favorite colorant, essential oils or herbs to the mixture.

Pour the finished mixture into clean container and seal tightly.

To use, pour small amount in the palm of your hand or apply it with a gentle upward motion. Allow the mixture to sit on your skin for 30-60 seconds before rinsing. This is also an excellent cleanser to add to your favorite scrubbing sacks. This is a soap mixture so always rinse your skin thoroughly when done washing.

Remember that everyone's skin reacts differently. You should test the products on a less sensitive area before using them. You should also remember that even natural products have side effects. The appendix gives the most common expected benefits and results of these ingredients. You should review these entries before trying any recipe.

Healing Cleanser

This is an excellent cleansing gel for both the face and the body. We use it whenever our skin is overstressed, irritated, or we just need a bit of skin help. The arrowroot powder helps to condition the skin aiding it in retaining moisture while promoting healing. The glycerin attracts moisture, promoting repair of the damage and helping to give a hydrated, supple look to the skin.

2 tbsp.	Abscess Root
2 cups	Distilled Water
1 tbsp.	Arrowroot Powder
1 tbsp.	Apple Cider Vinegar
2 tbsp.	Glycerin
	Emulsifier & Thickener as desired

Heat the water to a light boil. Remove the water from the heat and add the abscess root. Allow the mixture to steep for 4-6 hours until a dark tea has formed. Strain the plant parts from the liquid. The fluid will become the base for your recipe.

Re-heat the water until it is warm but not hot and add the powders. Stir the mixture until the powders are dissolved and the mixture begins to thicken. If mixture becomes thicker than desired, you may add additional water until you obtain the consistency you prefer.

Add the remaining ingredients and stir the cleanser gently until it is well blended.

While I do add herbs & oils that contain beneficial compounds, I typically do not add color or fragrance to any product designed for damaged skin because additives can cause the irritation to worsen. If you prefer something other than the natural color or scent, you can add your favorite colorant, essential oils, or herbs to the mixture.

Store the finished mixture in a tightly sealed container. A pump bottles work well with this base. To use, pump a pea sized drop into the palm of your hand and massage it into your skin using an upward motion. Allow the cleanser to sit on your skin for 30-60 seconds before rinsing. This is a soap mixture so always rinse your skin thoroughly when done washing.

Remember that everyone's skin reacts differently. You should test the products on a less sensitive area before using them. You should also remember that even natural products have side effects. The appendix gives the most common expected benefits and results of these ingredients. You should review these entries before trying any recipe.

Daily Damage Control Cleanser

This cleanser is mildly astringent with the juices helping to combat dryness while the honey acts to repair damage. The ingredients also aid in the prevention of new scales.

1 tbsp.	Red Clover
1 tsp.	Borax powder
¼ cup	Water

Heat the borax and water until they are just boiling. Remove the mixture from the heat and add the red clover. Allow the mixture to steep for 4-6 hours until a dark tea has formed. Strain the plant products from the liquid and add

2 tbsp.	Apple juice
2 tsp.	Aloe Vera Gel
1 tsp.	Evening Primrose Oil
1 tsp.	Tamanu Oil
	Emulsifier & Thickener as desired

Stir the cleanser gently until all of the ingredients are well blended.

This mixture will be slightly looser than the others will so you may wish to add a thickening agent for easier application.

This recipe has a lovely sweet smell and a pretty color but if you desire a specific color or fragrance, you may add your favorite colorant or essential oils or herbs to the mixture.

While I do add herbs & oils that contain beneficial compounds, I typically do not add color or fragrance to any product designed for damaged skin because additives can cause the irritation to worsen.

Store the finished mixture in a tightly sealed container. A pump bottles work well with this base. To use, pump a pea sized drop into the palm of your hand and massage it into your skin using an upward motion. Allow the cleanser to sit on your skin for 30-60 seconds before rinsing. This is a soap mixture so always rinse your skin thoroughly when done washing.

Remember that everyone's skin reacts differently. You should test the products on a less sensitive area before using them. You should also remember that even natural products have side effects. The appendix gives the most common expected benefits and results of these ingredients. You should review these entries before trying any recipe.

Sweet Radiance Cleanser

Even those who suffer from psoriasis can have a well-hydrated, radiant glow. I love to use this one whenever I need a refreshed look and best of all the cleanser acts to prevent future flares.

2 tbsp .	Plain Yogurt
1 tsp.	Honey – clover honey works best
1 tbsp.	Safflower Oil
1 tbsp.	Argon Oil
1 tbsp .	Fennel Oil
1 tbsp .	Rosewater (you may use Witch Hazel if desired)
	Emulsifier & Thickener as desired

Place all of the ingredients in a blender and mix well.

While I do add herbs & oils that contain beneficial compounds, I typically do not add color or fragrance to any product designed for damaged skin because additives can cause the irritation to worsen. This cleanser has a beautiful, light fragrance of its own, but if you desire a specific color or fragrance, you may add your favorite colorant or essential oils or herbs to the mixture

Spoon the mixture into a clean container and seal it tightly.

Refrigeration may lengthen the shelf life of the product. This recipe makes one or two applications. If you choose to enlarge the recipe, refrigeration is necessary.

To use, place a small amount of the paste in the palm of your hand and apply to your skin in an upward motion. Allow the cleanser to sit on the 30-60 seconds before rinsing. This is a soap mixture so always rinse your skin thoroughly when done washing.

Remember that everyone's skin reacts differently. You should test the products on a less sensitive area before using them. You should also remember that even natural products have side effects. The appendix gives the most common expected benefits and results of these ingredients. You should review these entries before trying any recipe.

Soothing Wash

This is one of the more soothing skin washes. It works best when skin irritation is the most severe. It helps to hydrate while easing the inflammation.

1 tbsp.	Marshmallow Root
1 cup	Warm Water

Marshmallow Root tends to respond best as a cold infusion. The water should be warm, not hot when you add the root. Place the mixture in a cool place and allow the root to steep for up to 24 hours. Stain the marshmallow root from the liquid. The liquid should be a bit thicker than a regular tea. Add

3 tsp.	Aloe Vera Gel
1 tsp.	Argon Oil
1 tsp.	Cajuput Oil
	Emulsifier & Thickener as desired

Stir the remaining ingredients into the marshmallow root liquid until they are well blended.

While I do add herbs & oils that contain beneficial compounds, I typically do not add color or fragrance to any product designed for damaged skin because additives can cause the irritation to worsen. If you prefer something other than the natural color or scent, you can add your favorite colorant, essential oils, or herbs to the mixture.

Pour the mixture into a clean, dry bottle with a tight fitting lid.

The mixture will separate if it is left standing so shake the cleanser well before each use.

Apply to the skin with a gentle upward motion. Allow the cleanser to sit on the skin for 30-60 seconds before rinsing. This is a soap mixture so always rinse your skin thoroughly when done washing.

Remember that everyone's skin reacts differently. You should test the products on a less sensitive area before using them. You should also remember that even natural products have side effects. The appendix gives the most common expected benefits and results of these ingredients. You should review these entries before trying any recipe.

Astringents & Toners

Astringents & Toners are an essential element to maintaining healthy skin. They work with your cleansers, serums, and lotions to help keep the skin clean, hydrated, and healthy. Astringents & toners help get rid of the residue that cleansers sometimes leave behind.

Astringents and toners also help to prevent future psoriasis outbreaks and to minimize the appearance of current outbreaks. You should select astringent and toner recipes that complement your other daily care regimen components.

Remember that everyone's skin reacts differently. You should test the products on a less sensitive area before using them. You should also remember that even natural products have side effects. The appendix gives the most common expected benefits and results of these ingredients. You should review these entries before trying any recipe.

Basic Astringent

This is a great basic astringent for every day needs. It also makes an excellent base for custom astringent products designed to suit your specific needs. You can use this astringent as the recipe shows if you wish. More commonly, this astringent is one that you will use as a base for customization. You should review the appendix ingredient listing and add the ingredients that best suit your skin care needs.

5 tbsp   Rosewater

You may substitute distilled water if preferred

1 tbsp   Witch Hazel

1/8 tsp   Borax Powder

Dissolve the borax in the rosewater. You may need to heat the rosewater slightly to help dissolve the borax powder. Do not boil the rosewater since this can cause some of the beneficial compound to be destroyed and will result in some evaporation.

Add the witch hazel and stir the mixture until it is well blended.

You may want to select ingredients from the appendix to strengthen the affect of the toner. You should decide what ingredients best suit your skin care goals and add them accordingly. You do not have to add any other compounds if you do not need enhanced treatments since this toner works very well alone.

While I do add herbs & oils that contain beneficial compounds, I typically do not add color or fragrance to any product designed for damaged skin because additives can cause the irritation to worsen. If you prefer something other than the natural color or scent, you can add your favorite colorant, essential oils, or herbs to the mixture.

Store the finished toner in an airtight container to prevent evaporation. Apply the toner to your skin using a clean cotton ball. Do not rinse this recipe from your skin. Allow the liquid to dry naturally and continue to work throughout the day. You can use moisturizer & makeup after the liquid has dried.

Remember that everyone's skin reacts differently. You should test the products on a less sensitive area before using them. You should also remember that even natural products have side effects. The appendix gives the most common expected benefits and results of these ingredients. You should review these entries before trying any recipe.

Juicy Juice Astringent

Juices from apples, cherries, plums or berries contain sorbitol. Sorbitol is a natural humectant that attracts moisture and provides a smooth texture. This is one of my favorite astringent products because it helps to keep my skin fresh, promotes a nice smooth, tight texture and supports healing of psoriasis scales.

½ cup   Juice of Choice

3 tbsp   Rosewater

1 tbsp.   Powdered Bladderwort

Heat the juice and rosewater lightly to encourage the bladderwort powder to dissolve. Blend all of the ingredients.

While I do add herbs & oils that contain beneficial compounds, I typically do not add color or fragrance to any product designed for damaged skin because additives can cause the irritation to worsen. If you prefer something other than the natural color or scent, you can add your favorite colorant, essential oils, or herbs to the mixture.

This recipe may separate so shake it well before each use. You may wish to store this recipe in the refrigerator to extend the shelf life. Do not rinse this recipe from your skin. Allow the liquid to dry naturally and continue to work throughout the day. You can use moisturizer & makeup after the liquid has dried.

Remember that everyone's skin reacts differently. You should test the products on a less sensitive area before using them. You should also remember that even natural products have side effects. The appendix gives the most common expected benefits and results of these ingredients. You should review these entries before trying any recipe.

Smoothing & Toning Astringent

This is an excellent toner to help smooth & tone overstressed skin while acting as both a preventative and treatment for psoriasis sufferers. It works equally well on the face and body.

1 cup	Distilled Water
½ tsp.	Spikenard
½ tsp.	Loosestrife
½ cup	Witch Hazel

Bring the water to a light boil and remove it from the heat. Add the flowers and leaves to the hot water. Steep the flowers & leaves in the water for up to 24 hours or until you achieve a nice dark brew. Strain the flowers and leaves from the fluid and discard the plant parts. The fluid will act as the base for your toner.

Stir witch hazel into the liquid base.

While I do add herbs & oils that contain beneficial compounds, I typically do not add color or fragrance to any product designed for damaged skin because additives can cause the irritation to worsen. If you prefer something other than the natural color or scent, you can add your favorite colorant, essential oils, or herbs to the mixture.

Pour the finished toner into your favorite spray or dispenser bottle. Seal the container tightly to prevent evaporation.

Apply the finished product to your skin using a cotton ball or spritzer.

Do not rinse this recipe from your skin. Allow the liquid to dry naturally and continue to work throughout the day. You can use moisturizer & makeup after the liquid has dried.

Remember that everyone's skin reacts differently. You should test the products on a less sensitive area before using them. You should also remember that even natural products have side effects. The appendix gives the most common expected benefits and results of these ingredients. You should review these entries before trying any recipe

Brightening Toner

This is an excellent toner to help wake up dull skin, speed healing, and minimize the appearance of the flakes associated with psoriasis. It works equally well on the face and body.

1 cup	Distilled Water
½ tsp.	Chaulmoogra
½ tsp.	Basil
½ cup	Orange Flower Water

Bring the water to a light boil and remove it from the heat. Add the chaulmoogra and basil to the hot water. Steep the mixture for up to 24 hours or until you achieve a nice dark brew. Strain the leaves from the fluid and discard the plant parts. The fluid will act as the base for your toner.

Stir the orange flower water into the liquid base.

While I do add herbs & oils that contain beneficial compounds, I typically do not add color or fragrance to any product designed for damaged skin because additives can cause the irritation to worsen. If you prefer something other than the natural color or scent, you can add your favorite colorant, essential oils, or herbs to the mixture.

Pour the finished toner into your favorite spray or dispenser bottle. Seal the container tightly to prevent evaporation.

Apply the finished product to your skin using a cotton ball or spritzer.

Do not rinse this recipe from your skin. Allow the liquid to dry naturally and continue to work throughout the day. You can use moisturizer & makeup after the liquid has dried.

Remember that everyone's skin reacts differently. You should test the products on a less sensitive area before using them. You should also remember that even natural products have side effects. The appendix gives the most common expected benefits and results of these ingredients. You should review these entries before trying any recipe

Healing Toner

Honey is one of my favorite skin care ingredients. It not only helps to soften the skin, it also has antibacterial and healing properties while the mallow helps to reduce the inflammation associated with psoriasis. This toner works well for anyone who has sensitive skin.

2 tbsp	Honey
4 tbsp	Strong Common Mallow Tea
4 tbsp	Rosewater

You can make the mallow tea using 1 tbsp. of mallow and ½-cup water. Bring the mixture to a boil until the fluid has been reduced by about ½ to ¼ cup. Mallow sometimes yields best as a cold infusion so you may wish to allow the mixture to sit overnight to obtain the highest benefit from the treatment. Strain the plant parts from the fluid.

Blend all of the ingredients directly into the container you will use as a dispenser.

While I do add herbs & oils that contain beneficial compounds, I typically do not add color or fragrance to any product designed for damaged skin because additives can cause the irritation to worsen. If you prefer something other than the natural color or scent, you can add your favorite colorant, essential oils, or herbs to the mixture.

The toner will be sticky at first. Aging helps to diminish the sticky quality. I like to age this toner for about 1 week before use but you can use it immediately if you wish.

Do not rinse this recipe from your skin. Allow the liquid to dry naturally and continue to work throughout the day. You can use moisturizer & makeup after the liquid has dried.

Remember that everyone's skin reacts differently. You should test the products on a less sensitive area before using them. You should also remember that even natural products have side effects. The appendix gives the most common expected benefits and results of these ingredients. You should review these entries before trying any recipe.

Cooling Toner

This tone is one of the most effective for alleviating itching skin, soothing inflammation and speeding healing while reducing the redness associated with healing scales. This toner has one of the cleanest scents and is a favorite of everyone in the house during the warmer months.

4 tbsp.	Camphor
¼ cup	Witch Hazel
¼ cup	Rosewater

Mix the ingredients until they are well blended.

While I do add herbs & oils that contain beneficial compounds, I typically do not add color or fragrance to any product designed for damaged skin because additives can cause the irritation to worsen. If you prefer something other than the natural color or scent, you can add your favorite colorant, essential oils, or herbs to the mixture.

Store the completed toner in an airtight container. You may wish to place the container in the refrigerator to increase the shelf life of the finished product.

Do not rinse this recipe from your skin. Allow the liquid to dry naturally and continue to work throughout the day. You can use moisturizer & makeup after the liquid has dried.

Remember that everyone's skin reacts differently. You should test the products on a less sensitive area before using them. You should also remember that even natural products have side effects. The appendix gives the most common expected benefits and results of these ingredients. You should review these entries before trying any recipe.

Gentle Astringent

Dealing with Psoriasis sometimes increases skin sensitivity making the products that we choose to use for cleaning especially important. Many of the more common treatments are harsh and can damage sensitive skin. This nice toner helps to promote clear, fresh looking skin without creating irritation.

4 tbsp	Rosewater
4 tbsp	Orange Flower Water
2 tbsp.	Aloe Vera Water
½ tsp.	Camphor

Pour the liquids directly into a spray bottle. Shake the bottle well to blend the ingredients.

While I do add herbs & oils that contain beneficial compounds, I typically do not add color or fragrance to any product designed for damaged skin because additives can cause the irritation to worsen. If you prefer something other than the natural color or scent, you can add your favorite colorant, essential oils, or herbs to the mixture.

Shake the completed toner well before each use. Do not rinse this recipe from your skin. Allow the liquid to dry naturally and continue to work throughout the day. You can use moisturizer & makeup after the liquid has dried.

Remember that everyone's skin reacts differently. You should test the products on a less sensitive area before using them. You should also remember that even natural products have side effects. The appendix gives the most common expected benefits and results of these ingredients. You should review these entries before trying any recipe.

Scar Reduction Toner

Flaking scales can create dark pigmentation spots on the skin. This is a nice toner to use on a regular basis to help reduce the appearance of light pitting and hyper-pigmentation while keeping the skin free of dirt, oils, and toxins.

4 tbsp	Rosewater
4 tbsp	Powdered Avens
4 tbsp.	Papaya Milk

Pour the ingredients directly into a spray bottle. Add the powdered Avens and shake the bottle until the ingredients are well blended. You may need to heat the ingredients a bit to help the powder dissolve.

While I do add herbs & oils that contain beneficial compounds, I typically do not add color or fragrance to any product designed for damaged skin because additives can cause the irritation to worsen. If you prefer something other than the natural color or scent, you can add your favorite colorant, essential oils, or herbs to the mixture.

Shake the completed toner well before each use. Do not rinse this recipe from your skin. Allow the liquid to dry naturally and continue to work throughout the day. You can use moisturizer & makeup after the liquid has dried.

Remember that everyone's skin reacts differently. You should test the products on a less sensitive area before using them. You should also remember that even natural products have side effects. The appendix gives the most common expected benefits and results of these ingredients. You should review these entries before trying any recipe.

CHAPTER

4

Mask & Wrap Treatments

Sometimes a deep treatment mask or wrap helps to maximize the benefits of daily care. At other times, deep treatments are necessary to start the treatment processes and remove obstacles that can interfere with your selected daily cleansing & moisturizing plans.

Mask treatments are designed to deliver concentrated benefits to a specific area helping to achieve results much more quickly. Masks should not be overused since they tend to be more concentrated and overuse can actually cause more damage than benefit.

Mask treatments are among the most customizable of all of the recipes in this book. Masks & Deep Treatments help to pamper your skin and prepare it for a daily regimen that will help you achieve healthy, beautiful skin. You should refer to the optional ingredient list to customize the deep treatment recipe, making one that suits your personal needs & desires.

While I do add herbs & oils that contain beneficial compounds, I typically do not add color or fragrance to any product designed for damaged skin because additives can cause the irritation to worsen. If you prefer something other than the natural color or scent, you can add your favorite colorant, essential oils, or herbs to the recipes.

Remember that everyone's skin reacts differently. You should test the products on a less sensitive area before using them. You should also remember that even natural products have side effects. The appendix gives the most common expected benefits and results of these ingredients. You should review these entries before trying any recipe.

Collagen Building Mask or Wrap

Gelatin is one of my favorite mask bases. It is not as drawing as clay and it helps to attract moisture to the skin while the other ingredients reduce irritation, itchiness, and redness associated with psoriasis.

½ cup	Gelatin – 1 packet
½ cup	Distilled Water
1 tsp.	Damask Rose Oil

Mix the gelatin and water until they are well blended.

Before the gelatin hardens, stir in the remaining ingredients.

The product will have its own natural scent and color, but if you desire a specific color to suit your needs or an aromatherapy benefit you may add your favorite colorant or essential oils to the recipe. While I do add herbs & oils that contain beneficial compounds, I typically do not add color or fragrance to any product designed for damaged skin because additives can cause the irritation to worsen.

To use, apply the mixture to your skin in an even coat.

Allow the mixture to soak into your skin for approximately 30 minutes or until the gelatin is completely dry.

Peel or rinse the mask from your skin.

Remember that everyone's skin reacts differently. You should test the products on a less sensitive area before using them. You should also remember that even natural products have side effects. The appendix gives the most common expected benefits and results of these ingredients. You should review these entries before trying any recipe.

Toning Wrap

This wrap is a one of my favorite recipes. It actually helps to reduce the appearance of psoriasis scales while toning the skin.

½ cup	Kaolin Clay
1 tbsp.	Henna Powder
2 tbsp.	Licorice Root
½ cup	Distilled Water
1 tsp.	Kukui Nut Oil
1 tsp.	Safflower Oil

Dissolve the powders in the liquid and then add the oil stirring until it is evenly distributed. The mixture will form a thick paste.

You do not want the mixture to be too wet since it may be difficult to apply. If it is too firm, add a few extra dashes of clay until it reaches the desired consistency. If it is too firm, you can add a few drops of water until you get the consistency you want.

The product will have its own natural scent and color, but if you desire a specific color to suit your needs or an aromatherapy benefit you may add your favorite colorant or essential oils to the recipe. While I do add herbs & oils that contain beneficial compounds, I typically do not add color or fragrance to any product designed for damaged skin because additives can cause the irritation to worsen.

To use, apply the mixture to your skin in an even coat.

Allow the mixture to soak into your skin for approximately 30 minutes or until the gelatin is completely dry.

Rinse the wrap from your skin and follow it with a healing moisturizing treatment.

Remember that everyone's skin reacts differently. You should test the products on a less sensitive area before using them. You should also remember that even natural products have side effects. The appendix gives the most common expected benefits and results of these ingredients. You should review these entries before trying any recipe.

Aloe Vera Healing Wrap

Aloe Vera is a wonderful treatment for many, many problems. Perhaps one of the best uses aloe is to sooth skin irritation while supporting collagen-building mechanisms. Safflower and Juniper are two of my favorite additives but you can select almost any other powder or oil from the appendix list to include in your personal healing wrap.

¼ cup	Powdered Clay – Kaolin works best
¼ cup	Aloe Vera Gel
1 tbsp.	Juniper Oil
1 tbsp.	Safflower Oil

Blend the oils and slowly add them to the aloe vera base stirring well to ensure that you have an even distribution.

Slowly stir in the clay until the mixture forms a thick paste. If the mixture is too dry, you can add a few drops of orange flower water until the desired consistency is obtained.

The product will have its own natural scent and color, but if you desire a specific color to suit your needs or an aromatherapy benefit you may add your favorite colorant or essential oils to the recipe. While I do add herbs & oils that contain beneficial compounds, I typically do not add color or fragrance to any product designed for damaged skin because additives can cause the irritation to worsen.

To use, apply the mixture to your skin in an even coat.

Allow the mixture to soak into your skin for approximately 30 minutes or until the clay is completely dry.

Rinse the wrap from your skin and follow it with a healing moisturizing treatment.

Remember that everyone's skin reacts differently. You should test the products on a less sensitive area before using them. You should also remember that even natural products have side effects. The appendix gives the most common expected benefits and results of these ingredients. You should review these entries before trying any recipe.

Deep Infusion Mask

Gelatin works wonders for attracting moisture and helping the additives in a mask recipe to infuse their benefits into the skin. This mask is wonderful for hydrating and brightening dull skin while giving it the nourishment it needs to reduce the severity of a psoriasis outbreak while helping to prevent future flares.

½ cup	Gelatin – 1 packet
½ cup	Distilled Water
½ tsp.	Phellodendron Powder
½ tsp.	Tamanu Oil

Mix the gelatin and water until they are well blended.

Before the gelatin hardens, stir in the remaining ingredients.

If the mixture is too thick, you can add a few drops of warm water until the mixture reaches your preferred consistency. If the mixture is too loose, allow the gelatin to solidify a bit longer before using the mask.

The product will have its own natural scent and color, but if you desire a specific color to suit your needs or an aromatherapy benefit you may add your favorite colorant or essential oils to the recipe. While I do add herbs & oils that contain beneficial compounds, I typically do not add color or fragrance to any product designed for damaged skin because additives can cause the irritation to worsen.

To use, apply the mixture to your skin in an even coat.

Allow the mixture to soak into your skin for approximately 30 minutes or until the gelatin is completely dry.

Peel or rinse the mask from your skin.

Remember that everyone's skin reacts differently. You should test the products on a less sensitive area before using them. You should also remember that even natural products have side effects. The appendix gives the most common expected benefits and results of these ingredients. You should review these entries before trying any recipe.

Soothing Mask

One of the hardest parts of dealing with psoriasis is resisting the urge to scratch the scales making the problem worse. This is a fantastic mask to reduce the itchiness associated with an outbreak while helping to minimize redness and speed healing. Henna comes in colored and colorless forms and you will want to be sure that you are using colorless henna powder unless you are hoping to make a sunless tanning product out of your wrap!

| ½ cup | Colorless Henna Powder |

½ cup   Colorless Henna Powder

¼ cup   Witch Hazel

¼ cup   Warm Distilled Water

2 tbsp.   Powdered Golden Seal

Stir the goldenseal and henna powders until they are well blended.

Slowly add the blended powders to the liquid until the ingredients form a thick paste. If the mixture is too liquid, you can add a bit more henna powder. If the mixture it too solid, you can add a few extra drops of witch hazel.

The product will have its own natural scent and color, but if you desire a specific color to suit your needs or an aromatherapy benefit you may add your favorite colorant or essential oils to the recipe. While I do add herbs & oils that contain beneficial compounds, I typically do not add color or fragrance to any product designed for damaged skin because additives can cause the irritation to worsen.

To use, apply the mixture to your skin in an even coat.

Allow the mixture to soak into your skin for approximately 30 minutes or until the gelatin is completely dry.

Rinse the mask from your skin and follow with a hydrating moisturizer.

Remember that everyone's skin reacts differently. You should test the products on a less sensitive area before using them. You should also remember that even natural products have side effects. The appendix gives the most common expected benefits and results of these ingredients. You should review these entries before trying any recipe.

Reversal Mask

This is one of my favorite masks to speed healing while reducing the itchiness and scales associated with a flare up. I prefer the kelp mask as a base, but you can add the active components to almost any mask base you prefer.

½ cup	Powdered Brown Kelp
1 tsp.	Powdered Little Mallow Root
½ cup	Distilled Water
½ tsp.	Evening Primrose Oil

Mix the powders and water until they are well blended.

Before the mixture hardens, stir in the oil.

If the powder is too dry and flaky, add a few extra drops of distilled water until the mask reaches the desired texture. If the mask is too moist, add a few extra dashes of clay until the mixture firms enough for easy application.

The product will have its own natural scent and color, but if you desire a specific color to suit your needs or an aromatherapy benefit you may add your favorite colorant or essential oils to the recipe. While I do add herbs & oils that contain beneficial compounds, I typically do not add color or fragrance to any product designed for damaged skin because additives can cause the irritation to worsen.

To use, apply the paste to your skin in an even coat.

Allow the mixture to soak into your skin for approximately 30 minutes or until it is completely dry.

Peel the mixture from the skin, rinse well, and pat the skin dry.

Remember that everyone's skin reacts differently. You should test the products on a less sensitive area before using them. You should also remember that even natural products have side effects. The appendix gives the most common expected benefits and results of these ingredients. You should review these entries before trying any recipe.

Serums

Healthy skin is not just about cleansing. Healthy skin is about creating the right mixture of cleanliness, hydration, and moisture. Serums & lotions are critical to the success of your skin care regimen.

Some areas of your skin may need additional serums and treatments to help combat the irritation created by other treatments, target specific problems, and reduce the number and severity of your psoriasis flares. Serums tend to be lightweight and thinner making applications to the face, scales, and smaller areas easier.

Serums are often oil-based treatments. This helps to maximize the benefits of the serum while minimizing the chance of doing inadvertent damage through the use of additives like thickening agents.

Lotions work much like serums but are traditionally thicker and heavier. While serums work well on the face and areas that have severe scaling, lotions tend to be a better choice for the rest of the body.

Remember that everyone's skin reacts differently. You should test the products on a less sensitive area before using them. You should also remember that even natural products have side effects. The appendix gives the most common expected benefits and results of these ingredients. You should review these entries before trying any recipe.

Healing Serum

This is a wonderful massage to use to stimulate healing of facial psoriasis or scales on other areas that are particularly sensitive.

4 tsp.	Almond Oil
1 tsp.	Safflower Oil
½ tsp.	Cade Oil
½ tsp.	Argon Oil
	Emulsifier & Thickener as desired

While I do add herbs & oils that contain beneficial compounds, I typically do not add color or fragrance to any product designed for damaged skin because additives can cause the irritation to worsen. If you prefer something other than the natural color or scent, you can add your favorite colorant, essential oils, or herbs to the mixture.

Gently blend the oils in a clean container. Store the mixture in a pump container that allows you to dispense 1 or 2 drops at a time. The oils may separate if allowed to sit so shake the mixture well before each use. Apply an even coat of the oils to the skin in the morning and at night. Do not rinse the mixture from the skin.

Remember that everyone's skin reacts differently. You should test the products on a less sensitive area before using them. You should also remember that even natural products have side effects. The appendix gives the most common expected benefits and results of these ingredients. You should review these entries before trying any recipe.

Sensitive Skin Serum

This serum works very well for sensitive skin. It also helps to reduce the appearance of a current flare while minimizing the likelihood of new psoriasis scaling.

2 tsp   Tamanu Oil

2 tsp   Safflower Oil

While I do add herbs & oils that contain beneficial compounds, I typically do not add color or fragrance to any product designed for damaged skin because additives can cause the irritation to worsen. If you prefer something other than the natural color or scent, you can add your favorite colorant, essential oils, or herbs to the mixture.

Gently blend the oils in a clean container. Store the mixture in a pump container that allows you to dispense 1 or 2 drops at a time. The oils may separate if allowed to sit so shake the mixture well before each use. Apply an even coat of the oils to the skin in the morning and at night. Do not rinse the mixture from the skin.

Remember that everyone's skin reacts differently. You should test the products on a less sensitive area before using them. You should also remember that even natural products have side effects. The appendix gives the most common expected benefits and results of these ingredients. You should review these entries before trying any recipe.

Hydrating Serum

Jojoba is an excellent base for serums since it is close to the skins natural oils and easily absorbed. This is my base facial serum for every day use and a favorite for treating dry, flaking patches. It is important to hydrate healthy skin but doubly important when psoriasis scales appear.

2 tsp	Jojoba Oil
2 tsp	Damask Rose Oil
1 tsp	Evening Primrose Oil
	Emulsifier & Thickener as desired

While I do add herbs & oils that contain beneficial compounds, I typically do not add color or fragrance to any product designed for damaged skin because additives can cause the irritation to worsen. If you prefer something other than the natural color or scent, you can add your favorite colorant, essential oils, or herbs to the mixture.

Gently blend the oils in a clean container. Store the mixture in a pump container that allows you to dispense 1 or 2 drops at a time. The oils may separate if allowed to sit so shake the mixture well before each use. Apply an even coat of the oils to the skin in the morning and at night. Do not rinse the mixture from the skin.

Remember that everyone's skin reacts differently. You should test the products on a less sensitive area before using them. You should also remember that even natural products have side effects. The appendix gives the most common expected benefits and results of these ingredients. You should review these entries before trying any recipe.

Soothing Serum

Itching, redness, and discomfort are all hallmarks of psoriasis flare up. This serum helps to tighten the skin while acting to combat symptoms.

5 tsp	Apricot Kernel Oil
1 tsp	Camphor Oil
1 tsp	Borage Seed Oil
	Emulsifier & Thickener as desired

While I do add herbs & oils that contain beneficial compounds, I typically do not add color or fragrance to any product designed for damaged skin because additives can cause the irritation to worsen. If you prefer something other than the natural color or scent, you can add your favorite colorant, essential oils, or herbs to the mixture.

Gently blend the oils in a clean container. Store the mixture in a pump container that allows you to dispense 1 or 2 drops at a time. The oils may separate if allowed to sit so shake the mixture well before each use. Apply an even coat of the oils to the skin in the morning and at night. Do not rinse the mixture from the skin.

Remember that everyone's skin reacts differently. You should test the products on a less sensitive area before using them. You should also remember that even natural products have side effects. The appendix gives the most common expected benefits and results of these ingredients. You should review these entries before trying any recipe.

Daily Toning Serum

This nice toning serum helps to tighten & refine the appearance of pores while giving the skin the boost it needs to speed healing of psoriasis scales.

2 tsp.	Sunflower Seed Oil
½ tsp.	Powdered Hyacinth Bulb
½ tsp.	Juniper Oil
	Emulsifier & Thickener as desired

While I do add herbs & oils that contain beneficial compounds, I typically do not add color or fragrance to any product designed for damaged skin because additives can cause the irritation to worsen. If you prefer something other than the natural color or scent, you can add your favorite colorant, essential oils, or herbs to the mixture.

Gently blend the oils in a clean container. Store the mixture in a pump container that allows you to dispense 1 or 2 drops at a time. The oils may separate if allowed to sit so shake the mixture well before each use. Apply an even coat of the oils to the skin in the morning and at night. Do not rinse the mixture from the skin.

Remember that everyone's skin reacts differently. You should test the products on a less sensitive area before using them. You should also remember that even natural products have side effects. The appendix gives the most common expected benefits and results of these ingredients. You should review these entries before trying any recipe.

Nighttime Healing Gel

This toning gel helps to reduce puffiness, plump the skin and speed healing all at once. This can be too much for those with especially sensitive skin so do a skin test before use. Aloe tends to leave a shiny residue behind when it dries so this makes a better nighttime treatment.

1 tbsp.	Aloe Vera Gel
¼ tsp.	Tamanu Oil
¼ tsp.	Kukui Nut Oil
	Emulsifier & Thickener as desired

While I do add herbs & oils that contain beneficial compounds, I typically do not add color or fragrance to any product designed for damaged skin because additives can cause the irritation to worsen. If you prefer something other than the natural color or scent, you can add your favorite colorant, essential oils, or herbs to the mixture.

Gently blend the oils in a clean container. Store the mixture in a pump container that allows you to dispense 1 or 2 drops at a time. The oils may separate if allowed to sit so shake the mixture well before each use. Apply an even coat of the oils to the skin in the morning and at night. Do not rinse the mixture from the skin.

Remember that everyone's skin reacts differently. You should test the products on a less sensitive area before using them. You should also remember that even natural products have side effects. The appendix gives the most common expected benefits and results of these ingredients. You should review these entries before trying any recipe.

Collagen Building Serum

Collagen loss is one aspect of post flare care that many people forget about. When scales flake off the skin, the area underneath is wounded. This can lead to pitting scars that occur when the collagen underlying the scales collapse. This oil helps to stimulate collagen production and should not be used on an active outbreak.

2 tsp.	Hazelnut Oil
1 tsp.	Borage Seed Oil
½ tsp.	Aloe Vera
	Emulsifier & Thickener as desired

While I do add herbs & oils that contain beneficial compounds, I typically do not add color or fragrance to any product designed for damaged skin because additives can cause the irritation to worsen. If you prefer something other than the natural color or scent, you can add your favorite colorant, essential oils, or herbs to the mixture.

Gently blend the oils in a clean container. Store the mixture in a pump container that allows you to dispense 1 or 2 drops at a time. The oils may separate if allowed to sit so shake the mixture well before each use. Apply an even coat of the oils to the skin in the morning and at night. Do not rinse the mixture from the skin.

Remember that everyone's skin reacts differently. You should test the products on a less sensitive area before using them. You should also remember that even natural products have side effects. The appendix gives the most common expected benefits and results of these ingredients. You should review these entries before trying any recipe.

Daily Dark Spot Reduction Serum

Sometimes psoriasis can leave dark marks behind when it heals. When these marks are pigmentation spots, you can help to fade them with the proper treatments. This is one of my favorites and best of all it works on freckles too! This serum should not be used on an active flare.

2 tsp.	Kukui Nut Oil
1 tsp.	Powdered Gotu Kola
½ tsp	Vitamin E Oil
½ tsp	Magnolia Oil
	Emulsifier & Thickener as desired

While I do add herbs & oils that contain beneficial compounds, I typically do not add color or fragrance to any product designed for damaged skin because additives can cause the irritation to worsen. If you prefer something other than the natural color or scent, you can add your favorite colorant, essential oils, or herbs to the mixture.

Gently blend the oils in a clean container. Store the mixture in a pump container that allows you to dispense 1 or 2 drops at a time. The oils may separate if allowed to sit so shake the mixture well before each use. Apply an even coat of the oils to the skin in the morning and at night. Do not rinse the mixture from the skin.

Remember that everyone's skin reacts differently. You should test the products on a less sensitive area before using them. You should also remember that even natural products have side effects. The appendix gives the most common expected benefits and results of these ingredients. You should review these entries before trying any recipe.

Nighttime Spot Reduction Gel

This gel is a nice alternative age spot reducing cream. It works best as a nighttime treatment because the gel tends to be a little shiny when it dries. This may not be as powerful as the Daily Dark Spot Reduction Serum but it also tends to be less irritating for those with sensitive skin.

2 tsp	Aloe Vera Gel
2 tsp	Powdered Asphodelus

While I do add herbs & oils that contain beneficial compounds, I typically do not add color or fragrance to any product designed for damaged skin because additives can cause the irritation to worsen. If you prefer something other than the natural color or scent, you can add your favorite colorant, essential oils, or herbs to the mixture.

Gently blend the oils in a clean container. Store the mixture in a pump container that allows you to dispense 1 or 2 drops at a time. The oils may separate if allowed to sit so shake the mixture well before each use. Apply an even coat of the oils to the skin in the morning and at night. Do not rinse the mixture from the skin.

Remember that everyone's skin reacts differently. You should test the products on a less sensitive area before using them. You should also remember that even natural products have side effects. The appendix gives the most common expected benefits and results of these ingredients. You should review these entries before trying any recipe.

CHAPTER 6

Lotions and Creams

Once you have clean and healthy looking skin, the next important focus to reducing the severity, number, and duration of psoriasis outbreaks is moisture. Your skin needs moisture to look its best and those who suffer from psoriasis often forget that hydration is critical to reducing the severity and duration of a flare.

The basic ingredients in moisturizing products are oil and water. Most creams also contain an emulsifier.

An emulsifier is a waxy substance that aids in keeping oil and water from separating. If you choose not to use an emulsifier, the creams and lotions you create will provide the same benefits but the components may separate when the product is left to sit. To correct this separation, shake the skin care product well before applying. This will serve to combine the ingredients and is an effective solution if you don't want an emulsifier in your mixture.

I typically do not use an emulsifier in my psoriasis care recipes. Additives can aggravate psoriasis and this irritation can lengthen the duration of an flare.

I do sometimes use a thickening agent to help make the lotions easier to apply. There are a few nice thickening agents listed in the appendix relating to optional ingredients. Some of the recipes already contain a beneficial thickening agent. Before modifying the recipe to include a thickening agent or an emulsifier, you should remember that these ingredients also have an affect on the skin. You should review the expected benefits, side effects, and warnings before selecting the one that might work best for your particular needs.

These recipes are ones that I use for lotions and creams that will be primarily applied to the body. Serums tend to be my go to option for the face and neck area. You should consider which ones will best suit your facial and body care needs and then choose the serum or lotion recipe that will work best for you.

Remember that everyone's skin reacts differently. You should test the products on a less sensitive area before using them. You should also remember that even natural products have side effects. The appendix gives the most common expected benefits and results of these ingredients. You should review these entries before trying any recipe.

Healing Lotion

This is an effective lotion for the body. It infuses the skin with various toning and emollient components while speed healing of psoriasis scales.

1 tbsp.   Loosestrife

¼ cup   Distilled Water

Heat the water until it reaches a light boil. Pour the boiling water over the loosestrife and allow the mixture to soak overnight. Drain the loosestrife from the liquid and discard the plant product. The liquid will act as the base for your recipe.

2 tbsp.   Grated Beeswax

1 tbsp.   Aloe Vera Gel

1 tsp.   Kukui Nut oil

1 tbsp.   Jojoba Oil

Combine beeswax and oils in a microwave safe dish and heat on medium for approximately 25 seconds or use a double boiler to bring the mixture to about 90 degrees.

Remove the mixture from the heat, stir it well and set it aside to cool slightly to about 70 degrees.

2 tbsp.   Aluminum Sulfate

3 tbsp.   Orange Flower Water

                Emulsifier & Thickener as desired

Use only *USP Grade for Cosmetic Use* aluminum sulfates.

Use only plastic or ceramic pans and utensils since aluminum sulfate can react with metals.

Dissolve the aluminum sulfate in the witch hazel and orange flower water.

Add the liquid and stir the mixture until it is well blended.

Slowly pour the liquid solution into the oil base stirring well.

The mixture will foam slightly as you stir.

The product will have its own natural scent and color, but if you desire a specific color to suit your needs or an aromatherapy benefit you may add your favorite colorant or essential oils to the recipe. While I do add herbs & oils that contain beneficial compounds, I typically do not add color or fragrance to any product designed for damaged skin because additives can cause the irritation to worsen.

Spoon the finished lotion into a clean container with a tight fitting lid. Allow the mixture to cool completely before use.

Massage the lotion in to the skin twice daily for the most beneficial results.

Remember that everyone's skin reacts differently. You should test the products on a less sensitive area before using them. You should also remember that even natural products have side effects. The appendix gives the most common expected benefits and results of these ingredients. You should review these entries before trying any recipe.

Scale Smoothing Lotion

This lovely light lotion is great for year round care. It helps to reduce the flaking associated with psoriasis scales while smoothing the skin around the outbreak leaving behind a supple and smooth texture. The natural humectant qualities of the glycerin attract moisture to provide a softening quality that helps to speed the healing of the outbreak while minimizing the likelihood of new scale formation.

3 tbsp.	Glycerin
3 tbsp.	Powdered Hyacinth Bulb
¼ cup	Kukui Nut Oil
¼ cup	Water
	Emulsifier & Thickener as desired

Mix all of the ingredients in a microwave safe dish and heat for approximately 1 minute until the mixture just begins to boil. Stir the mixture every 20-25 seconds during heating. You may also heat the mixture to a light boil in a double broiler.

The product will have its own natural scent and color, but if you desire a specific color to suit your needs or an aromatherapy benefit you may add your favorite colorant or essential oils to the recipe. While I do add herbs & oils that contain beneficial compounds, I typically do not add color or fragrance to any product designed for damaged skin because additives can cause the irritation to worsen. If you prefer something other than the natural color or scent, you can add your favorite colorant, essential oils, or herbs to the mixture.

Pour the finished lotion into a clean container and seal it tightly. Allow the lotion to cool completely before use.

To use pump or pour a small amount into the palm of your hand and massage gently into the skin. This lotion is more gel like so you will need to use care until you learn to manage the application.

Remember that everyone's skin reacts differently. You should test the products on a less sensitive area before using them. You should also remember that even natural products have side effects. The appendix gives the most common expected benefits and results of these ingredients. You should review these entries before trying any recipe.

Reduction Lotion

We call this the reduction lotion because it acts to reduce the appearance of scales, the itchiness of an outbreak, and the likelihood of a future outbreak.

2 tbsp.	Grated Beeswax
2 tbsp.	Evening Primrose Oil
1 tbsp.	Borage Seed Oil
¼ cup	Safflower Oil
¼ cup	Juice (pear, apple, cherry, plum or berry)
2 tbsp.	Rose Water
	Emulsifier & Thickener as desired

Place the beeswax and oils in a microwave safe dish and heat on medium approximately 25 seconds or use a double broiler to liquefy the mixture bringing it to approximately 90 degrees Fahrenheit. Remove the mixture from the heat and allow it to cool to approximately 70 degrees.

Combine the remaining ingredients in another dish.

Pour the juice mixture into the oil mixture and stir until well blended.

I love the natural smells and colors of this recipe and can alter the final product by changing the type of juice I use.

While I do add herbs & oils that contain beneficial compounds, I typically do not add color or fragrance to any product designed for damaged skin because additives can cause the irritation to worsen. If you prefer something other than the natural color or scent, you can add your favorite colorant, essential oils, or herbs to the mixture.

Allow the recipe to cool before use. The mixture will thicken as it cools.

Remember that everyone's skin reacts differently. You should test the products on a less sensitive area before using them. You should also remember that even natural products have side effects. The appendix gives the most common expected benefits and results of these ingredients. You should review these entries before trying any recipe.

Deep Hydration Lotion

Skin, especially skin suffering from a psoriasis flare up doesn't just need moisture on the surface it needs moisture deep down under the surface. Hydrating washes, lotions and treatments provide the benefit of total moisture infusion. This lotion is great for deep hydration and can be used daily to provide a supple, healthy appearance to skin.

2 tbsp.   Dried Chamomile Leaves

½ cup   Distilled Water

Heat the water until it is just boiling. Remove the water from the heat and pour it over the chamomile leaves. Allow the mixture to steep at least 6 hours until a darker tea is created. Strain the leaves from the tea and discard them. The liquid will act as your lotion base. Add

1 tsp.   Baking Soda

3 tbsp.   Glycerin

Combine the baking soda and glycerin with the chamomile water in a microwave safe dish. Heat on medium until the mixture just reaches boiling approximately 1 minute.

3 tbsp.   Stearic Acid Powder

¼ cup   Jojoba Oil

                Emulsifier & Thickener as desired

In another dish, combine the oils and stearic acid. Heat them on medium in the microwave for about 30 seconds until the liquid runs clear or in a double broiler until the mixture reaches about 90 degrees.

½ cup Carrot Juice

Add the carrot juice to the chamomile tea mixture and stir gently.

Slowly pour the chamomile mixture into the oil base.

The mixture will foam as it is mixed.

Stir gently to combine all of the ingredients.

Allow mixture to cool.

The mixture will have a golden orange color and a delicate fragrance. If you desire a personalized fragrance or color, you may add food coloring or your favorite essential oils to the mixture as it cools. While I do add herbs & oils that contain beneficial compounds, I typically do not add color or fragrance to any product designed for damaged skin because additives can cause the irritation to worsen. If you prefer something other than the natural color or scent, you can add your favorite colorant, essential oils, or herbs to the mixture.

Pour the lotion into a clean container and allow it to cool completely.

The mixture will thicken as it stands. Tightly seal the container.

This lotion will not keep as long as some others because of the juices. It may be stored in the refrigerator to lengthen the shelf life.

Remember that everyone's skin reacts differently. You should test the products on a less sensitive area before using them. You should also remember that even natural products have side effects. The appendix gives the most common expected benefits and results of these ingredients. You should review these entries before trying any recipe.

Daily Healing Lotion

Daily care is essential for healthy looking skin, for healing current scaling, and for minimizing the likelihood of future outbreaks. This is a nice general lotion for every day use.

¼ cup	Almond Oil
¼ cup	Safflower Oil
3 tbsp.	Stearic Acid Powder
1 tbsp.	Camphor
1 tbsp.	Baobab Oil
1 tbsp.	Tamanu Oil
2-3 drops	Tincture of Benzoin
	Emulsifier & Thickener as desired

Heat the almond oil, safflower oil, and stearic acid in the microwave on medium heat until mixture turns golden and foamy – approximately 35 seconds. You can also heat the mixture in a double broiler to approximately 90 degrees.

Remove the oils from the heat and set them aside to cool to about 70 degrees.

Combine remaining ingredients in another dish.

Whip the mixture with a whisk or in a blender until it foams slightly and all ingredients are well blended.

While I do add herbs & oils that contain beneficial compounds, I typically do not add color or fragrance to any product designed for damaged skin because additives can cause the irritation to worsen. If you prefer something other than the natural color or scent, you can add your favorite colorant, essential oils, or herbs to the mixture.

Pour the lotion into a clean container and allow it to cool. The lotion will thicken as it cools.

Remember that everyone's skin reacts differently. You should test the products on a less sensitive area before using them. You should also remember that even natural products have side effects. The appendix gives the most common expected benefits and results of these ingredients. You should review these entries before trying any recipe.

Daily Preventative Lotion

Daily prevention is one of the most important aspects of psoriasis care. Psoriasis is partially genetic but it also depends on triggers. This lotion helps to minimize some of the environmental triggers that can cause a flare while maximizing your body's ability to prevent future outbreaks.

2 tbsp.	Grated Beeswax

1 tbsp.	Cajuput Oil

Place the beeswax in a microwave safe dish and heat on medium approximately 25 seconds or use a double broiler to melt the beeswax bringing it to about 90 degrees. Remove the beeswax from the heat and allow it to cool slightly to about 70 degrees.

3 tbsp.	Powdered Holly Leaved Barberry

¼ tsp.	Borax Powder

Slowly add the borax mixture to the beeswax syrup.

¼ cup	Safflower Oil
	Emulsifier & Thickener as desired

Add the remaining ingredients and stir until they are well until they are well mixed.

While I do add herbs & oils that contain beneficial compounds, I typically do not add color or fragrance to any product designed for damaged skin because additives can cause the irritation to worsen. If you prefer something other than the natural color or scent, you can add your favorite colorant, essential oils, or herbs to the mixture.

Pour the lotion into a clean container and allow it to cool completely.

The mixture will thicken as it stands. Tightly seal the container.

Remember that everyone's skin reacts differently. You should test the products on a less sensitive area before using them. You should also remember that even natural products have side effects. The appendix gives the most common expected benefits and results of these ingredients. You should review these entries before trying any recipe.

Nourishing Daily Lotion

Well-nourished skin is beautiful skin and nourishing skin that suffers from psoriasis is twice as important. This lotion is full of compounds that are vital for nourished, healthy skin as well as compounds to help speed healing of scales. The lotion is light enough for every day use.

½ cup	Apricot Kernel Oil

1 tbsp.	Grated Beeswax

1 tbsp.	Almond Oil

Combine the oils and beeswax in a microwave safe dish and heat on medium for about 25 seconds or until the liquids melt to a consistency similar to syrup. You can also use a double broiler to heat the oils & wax to approximately 90 degrees.

Remove the mixture from the heat and set it aside to cool slightly to approximately 70 degrees Fahrenheit.

¼ tsp.	Borax Powder

½ cup	Water

Emulsifier & Thickener as desired

Dissolve the borax powder in the water. You may need to heat the water slightly to help dissolve the crystals.

Slowly add the borax mixture to the beeswax syrup.

You should use a wire whisk or a blender to ensure the ingredients are well mixed.

While I do add herbs & oils that contain beneficial compounds, I typically do not add color or fragrance to any product designed for damaged or sensitive skin because additives can cause the irritation to worsen. If you prefer something other than the natural color or scent, you can add your favorite colorant, essential oils, or herbs to the mixture.

Spoon the finished liquid into a clean container with a tight fitting lid. Allow the mixture to cool completely before use.

Massage the lotion in to the skin twice daily for the most beneficial results.

Remember that everyone's skin reacts differently. You should test the products on a less sensitive area before using them. You should also remember that even natural products have side effects. The appendix gives the most common expected benefits and results of these ingredients. You should review these entries before trying any recipe.

Remember that everyone's skin reacts differently. You should test the products on a less sensitive area before using them. You should also remember that even natural products have side effects. The appendix gives the most common expected benefits and results of these ingredients. You should review these entries before trying any recipe.

Deep Healing Cream

This is a deep penetrating cream that I use all over but truly love the most when skin needs extra healing. Beyond the penetration, the treatment leaves a protective film on the skin that helps prevent drying that can cause extra flaking in psoriasis scales. We like to make a heat pack out of this when an outbreak is especially bad by applying a thicker layer of the cream and then covering the treated area with plastic to let the oils really penetrate the skin.

½ cup	Safflower Oil
¼ cup	Wheat Germ Oil
2 tbsp.	Grated Beeswax
1 tbsp.	Powdered Golden Seal
1 tbsp.	Powdered Henna
	Emulsifier & Thickener as desired

Heat the oils and beeswax for approximately 25 seconds on medium in the microwave or until they form a thick syrup. You an also heat the ingredients to approximately 90 degrees Fahrenheit using a double broiler.

Remove the mixture from the heat and allow it to cool, stirring occasionally to prevent separation during the cooling stage.

While I do add herbs & oils that contain beneficial compounds, I typically do not add color or fragrance to any product designed for damaged skin because additives can cause the irritation to worsen. If you prefer something other than the natural color or scent, you can add your favorite colorant, essential oils, or herbs to the mixture.

Store the lotion in a clean container with a tight fitting lid.

To use, apply the lotion directly to the desired area and massage gently.

For a deeper conditioning action, heat the mixture slightly under warm water and apply a thick coat to desired areas. Cover the areas with saran wrap or a plastic bag and allow the mixture to penetrate the skin for 10-15 minutes.

Wipe remaining lotion from skin, but do not rinse the protective film off the skin.

Remember that everyone's skin reacts differently. You should test the products on a less sensitive area before using them. You should also remember that even natural products have side effects. The appendix gives the most common expected benefits and results of these ingredients. You should review these entries before trying any recipe.

CHAPTER 7

Mineral Makeup

Once your skin is clean, treated, and hydrated you may want to add makeup to enhance your overall appearance. Selecting a makeup can be a tough decision for those whose skin is prone to environmentally reactive psoriasis. You certainly do not want to select a makeup that is going to undo all that you have achieved through selective skin treatments. Facial scaling is also one of the hardest things to deal with about psoriasis. One solution that is becoming a popular choice among people with all types of skin but especially those who suffer from a condition like psoriasis is mineral makeup.

Mineral make up has been used for hundreds, even thousands of years across the globe. Over the last few years, interest in this natural skin colorant has undergone a tremendous boost. Many companies have developed lines of mineral makeup. Each touts the benefits of their line over the next. Whether one is better than another is a matter of opinion and I am not going to express mine here!

What I am going to do is tell you a few of the benefits all of these lines (and homemade mineral makeup) offer to you. Then, I will show you the recipe that I use to make mineral make up at home for myself, my daughter, my daughter's classmates and friends and even some of my friends and family. I like the make up that I make at home, love that I can feel comfortable having 'girl's day' with my 9 year old and her friends without worrying that I am ruining their skin, and especially love that it costs me pennies to make a years supply of makeup for everyone!

Mineral makeup is a wholly natural make up product created mostly from powdered minerals. The benefits of mineral make up are numerous but the most influential factor to most people is that it is 100% natural.

BENEFITS:

Mineral makeup is made from zinc and titanium dioxide so it is a natural sunscreen. Depending on how much you use SPF can range from 10 to 20.

Mineral makeup is typically water resistant. That is not to say waterproof but it does last much better while swimming or during water sports than many other make up products.

Mineral makeup is long-lasting, bearing up better to long days, outdoor activity, and even naps than more traditional make up products.

Mineral makeup contains ingredients that have special properties of their own. In addition to offering a natural sunscreen, you receive the side-benefits of each ingredient. If you look at the recipe for mineral base, you will see that zinc oxide is a main component. Zinc oxide has natural anti-inflammatory properties so the make up you make with zinc oxide will too!

When applied correctly, the coverage offered by mineral make up is lightweight and complete. This makes it perfect for all skin types – from young to old, oily to dry and everything in between.

Mineral make up is non-comedogenic and (unless you add oils to the recipe) oil free! This means it is less harmful and irritating to your skin. Some makers say it is so clean you can even sleep in it!

Mineral make up is all-natural and the ingredients (unless you add oils to the recipe) do not go bad. That means you do not have to add any preservatives to the mix making it healthier and more natural than the next makeup!

Mineral make up is fast and easy to apply.

Mineral make up is VERY inexpensive to make at home.

Base or Foundation

Base or foundation is applied all over the face to create a smooth texture, even skin tone, and flawless finish.

4 tsp. Micronized Titanium Dioxide

1 ½ tsp. Bismuth Oxychloride

2 tsp. Zinc Oxide – Low Micron

½ tsp. Magnesium Stearate

Mix base ingredients by blending well. You can use a mortar / pestle, metal spoon and bowl, or food processor to blend the ingredients.

Slowly add the pigment colorant to the mix.

+/- to preference

¼ tsp. Yellow Iron Oxide

Pinch Brown Iron Oxide

Pinch Red Iron Oxide

½ tsp. Sericite Mica - matte or translucent finish to suit final goals

You can change the tint of the final product to suit your skin tone and color preferences.

For darker shades, add more of any of the iron oxides.

For lighter shades, add more titanium dioxide or some serecite mica.

Some people have reported that Bismuth Oxychloride causes irritation and redness. If you have sensitive skin or develop a reaction to the recipe, you may try using less or no Bismuth Oxychloride in your recipe.

Some people might want to experiment with different color additives to correct or address certain problems. You could start with:

Yellow Oxide brightens dull complexions and counteracts redness.

Chromium Oxide Green counters redness from seborrhea, acne, or irritated skin.

Ultramarine Violet counters yellow or sallow skin tones; minimizes yellowish bruises.

Ultramarine Blue counters orange tones that may result from sunless tanning products.

LIQUID APPLICATION – some people prefer a bit more moisture in their makeup or like a liquid application more than a dry application. We make a liquid application by adding the powder mixture to our preferred moisturizer. The consistency of the liquid application is entirely a matter of preference. You will want to experiment by slowly adding the mineral mixture to your favorite moisturizer until you achieve the consistency and coverage amount you desire. The consistency ranges from full coverage matt to a lightweight tinted moisturizer.

Mineral Veil – Finish Powder

Mineral Veil is also called a finish powder and gives the face a translucent glow. It is applied on top of all other makeup.

3 tsp. Sericite Mica – Matte

1 tsp. Corn Starch

½ tsp. Boron Nitrate

½ tsp. Magnesium Stearate

Mix base ingredients by blending well. You can use a mortar / pestle, metal spoon and bowl, or food processor to blend the ingredients.

Slowly add the pigment colorant to the mix.

+/- to preference

Pinch Yellow Iron Oxide

Pinch Pink

Pinch Brown Iron Oxide

You can change the tint of the final product to suit your skin tone and color preferences.

For darker shades, add more of any of the iron oxides.

For lighter shades, add more Corn Starch.

Concealer

A concealer is similar to a foundation in composition with a few simple modifications. Concealer tends to be a couple of shades lighter than your foundation, provides more coverage and is more matte in finish.

½ tbsp. Micronized Titanium Dioxide

½ tbsp. Seracite Mica – Matte

¼ tbsp. Magnesium Stearate

Mix base ingredients by blending well. You can use a mortar / pestle, metal spoon and bowl, or food processor to blend the ingredients.

Slowly add the pigment colorant to the mix.

+/- to preference

1/16 tbsp. Yellow Iron Oxide

Pinch Red or Orange Iron Oxide

You can change the tint of the final product to suit your skin tone and color preferences.

For darker shades, add more of any of the iron oxides.

For lighter shades, add more titanium dioxide or some serecite mica.

Some people might want to experiment with different color additives to correct or address certain problems. You could start with:

Yellow Oxide brightens dull complexions or counteracts redness.

Chromium Green counters redness from seborrhea, acne, or irritated skin.

Ultramarine Violet counters yellow or sallow skin tones; minimizes yellowish bruises.

Ultramarine Blue counters orange tones that may result from sunless tanning products.

LIQUID APPLICATION - Some people prefer a bit more moisture in their makeup or like a liquid application more than a dry application. We make a liquid application by adding the powder mixture to our preferred moisturizer. The consistency of the liquid application is entirely a matter of preference. You will want to experiment by slowly adding the powder mixture to your favorite moisturizer until you achieve the consistency and coverage amount you desire.

Concealer often needs to be a bit heavier in weight. To create a heavier blend, you may want to try adding more mineral to the moisturizer or use a very heavy moisturizer as the base.

APPLICATION – DRY - To apply concealer in dry or powder form, first apply your foundation then use a small brush to apply the concealer directly to problem areas. Use a larger "Kabuki" brush to blend.

APPLICATION – WET - To apply concealer wet, put a small amount in the palm of your hand, add a small amount of water or moisturizer as desired, and apply with a brush or a sponge to problem areas. By applying wet, you can target larger problem areas. Allow concealer to dry after application. Apply powdered foundation over the concealer to blend and finish.

Bronzer

A bronzer gives extra color where the sun hits the face. The sun leaves a bronze or rosy hue behind. The bronzer gives you the ability to infuse a fresh, healthy glow to your skin without the dangers of spending the day in the sun.

2 tsp. Micronized Titanium Dioxide

1/3 tsp. Magnesium Stearate

Mix base ingredients by blending well. You can use a mortar / pestle, metal spoon and bowl, or food processor to blend the ingredients.

Slowly add the pigment colorant to the mix.

+/- to preference

½ tsp. Yellow Iron Oxide

½ tsp. Brown Iron Oxide

½ tsp. Red Iron Oxide

1 tsp. Sericite Mica – pearl finish

½ tsp. Bronze mica

You can change the tint of the final product to suit your skin tone and color preferences.

For darker shades, add more of any of the iron oxides.

For lighter shades, add more titanium dioxide or serecite mica.

Eye Shadow

Eye Shadow is used to give extra attention to the eyes.

1 tbsp. Micronized Titanium Dioxide

½ tsp. Magnesium Stearate

1 tsp. Sericite Mica – Pearl or Matte as preferred

Pearl Sericite will give you a shimmer effect eye shadow

Matte Sericite will give you a low luster eye shadow

Mix base ingredients by blending well. You can use a mortar / pestle, metal spoon and bowl, or food processor to blend the ingredients.

Slowly add the pigment colorant to the mix.

+/- to preference

½ tsp. Iron Oxide color of your choice

Start with ½ tsp and increase until desired color is obtained

We enjoy mixing multiple colors to attain a shadow that is specific to us. If you custom mix your shadow to your personal preference – DO NOT forget to write down what you did so you can repeat it later.

You can change the tint of the final product to suit your skin tone and color preferences.

For darker shades, add more of any of the iron oxides.

For lighter shades, add more titanium dioxide or some sericite mica.

Blush

Blush is used to accent the cheekbones and provide a healthy color to the face.

2 ¾ tsp. Sericite Mica

1/4 tsp. Micronized Titanium Dioxide

1/16 tsp. Arrowroot Powder

Mix base ingredients by blending well. You can use a mortar / pestle, metal spoon and bowl, or food processor to blend the ingredients.

Slowly add the pigment colorant to the mix.

+/- to preference

1/16 tsp. Red Iron Oxide

Start with 1/16 tsp and increase until desired color is obtained

We enjoy mixing multiple colors to attain a shadow that is specific to us. If you custom mix your shadow to your personal preference – DO NOT forget to write down what you did so you can repeat it later.

CHAPTER

8

Detoxification Teas

It is possible that there is a link between diet and the number and severity of psoriasis flares. It is believed that leaving certain items out of your diet might help to control your psoriasis. It is also possible that ingesting certain herbs may help to prevent flares or minimize the duration and severity of active psoriasis.

Herbalists have used herbal supplements for thousands of years to treat a variety of conditions. Research is constantly being conducted to determine the potential benefits of herbal supplements in relationship to psoriasis.

The following pages illustrate some herbal supplements that have been used as preventative or treatment options by for psoriasis. These herbal supplements are provided for informational purposes only. Nothing in this recipe guide is intended to substitute for the medical expertise and advice of your primary health care provider.

You should discuss any decisions about treatment or care with your health care provider. The information contained within this guide is believed to be accurate at the time of writing but research is being undertaken daily and new information, potential benefits, or side effects may be discovered that conflict with the materials contained in this guide.

No product, service, or therapy is endorsed by the author, publisher, or other individual associated with the creation of this material. The reader should remember that the U.S. Food and Drug Administration (FDA) have not evaluated herbal supplements. The items listed are not intended to diagnose, treat, cure, or prevent any disease.

Using any medication whether prescription, over the counter, or herbal in nature may have a marked effect on your health and each medicine may interact with others. Tell your health care provider about any complementary, supplemental, or alternative practices you use including dietary supplements, herbals, or oils.

Herbs and oils do have a noticeable affect on the human body. The expected action of many herbs and oils is based on traditional use and observation. Laboratory studies have been conducted to confirm the expected affect of some traditionally used herbs and oils but others have not been well researched. Most dietary supplements, herbs, and oils have not been researched for use by pregnant women, nursing women, or children.

Each person's needs and correct dosage will vary depending on a variety of factors. You should discuss your specific needs and best dosage with our physician or qualified herbalist.

Teas & Infusions
Teas and infusions are two of the most common methods of using herbal supplements. Making a natural tea or infusion allows you to obtain the benefits of the plants compounds while enjoying a variety of flavor sensations.

Infusions are not just for ingesting. You can use an infusion in the bath, in creams or lotions, as a wash, for cleaning, or for almost any other activity that can benefit from the compounds contained in the plants.

An infusion is made using the soft plant parts. These are parts like the flower or leaf.

You will need to decide the source of the water you will use to make your tea or infusion. Filtered water, spring water, and rainwater are all good sources. The primary concern with water is to ensure it has as few contaminates as possible.

You will want to choose a teapot or kettle for heating water that is not going to degrade and release chemicals into the final product. Glass, stainless steel, and ceramic are all common choices.

Warm the water to boiling in the kettle and then remove the water from the heat.

You will want to get a tea ball to contain your plant parts or tea strainer to help you remove the plant parts from the finished drink.

Tea balls tend to keep the plant parts together and leave far fewer 'clumps' in the finished drink but they also tend to compress the plant parts and make releasing the beneficial compounds more difficult.

Tea strainers allow the plant parts to move freely, releasing more of their compounds but also tend to allow small plant parts to escape into the finished drink.

Either option works well and the one that you choose will be based on your personal preference and needs.

You will choose the plant or combination of plant parts that provide the benefits you want from a supplement. These will vary greatly between people. You can even add a base tea just for the flavor! Regardless of the type of plants you are using, you will need between ¾ and 1 teaspoon of dried plant product per cup of liquid.

If you have not crumbled the plant parts before, you will want to break them into smaller pieces now. This gives the water more access to the plant parts and helps the compounds to release more easily.

You can add the dried pieces directly to your kettle as long as it has been removed from the heat source or place them in a cup and pour the water from the kettle on top.

Placing the herbs into the kettle, whether loose or in the tea ball, helps to prevent the oils from evaporating during steeping but also leaves residue behind that may be interfere with the next supplement you make if you do not clean the kettle well after each use.

Pouring the water over the leaves in the cup allows more of the beneficial compounds to escape during evaporation but helps to prevent cross contamination between supplement usages.

Either method of getting plant parts into contact with the water works and you should choose the option that suits you the best.

Allow the leaves to steep in the water for between 5 minutes and 6 hours depending on the supplement you are trying to create.

Once your drink is steeped to your desired strength, remove the plant parts from the liquid, flavor to taste and enjoy.

Cold Infusion

Many plants release their compounds best to warm water. Occasionally you may want to use a plant that does not release as well to heat. Some plants that are high in mucilage content or bitter compounds seem to do better when the compounds are infused in cold fluid.

A cold infusion is made by soaking the selected plant parts in room temperature or cooler liquid instead of hot water. You do not need to limit yourself to water. Some cold infusions are made with milk, juices, or another preferred liquid.

You will use the same proportions of plant parts and liquid as you do for a hot infusion. You will prepare the plant parts following the same processes. You will even consume the cold infusion the same way that you do a hot infusion. The two major differences when making a cold infusion are that you will use cold water, milk, or another liquid instead of hot and that you will allow the plant parts to steep for a longer period than you do with a warm infusion.

Angelica

Angelica root is believed to be a detoxifier and is traditionally used to cleanse the blood and combat psoriasis.

Part Used:
Root, Seeds, Stalks

Side Effects:
Angelica is not for use by women who are pregnant or nursing. Angelica is a strong emmanagogue and can cause a miscarriage.

Angelica should be used with caution as large doses can negatively affect blood pressure, heart, and respiration. Angelica should only be considered for internal use after consultation with a physician or qualified herbalist.

Angelica fruits can cause sun sensitivity in some individuals.

Angelia oils can irritate the skin and mucus membranes.

Additional uses and side effects may exist but further research is necessary to determine the exact properties and effects of use.

General:
Angelica can be found growing in temperate zones along running streams & rivers. Angelica prefers dense shade and moist soil. Angelica is often supplied as a fluid extract at a rate of 1:1 with 1 teaspoon of the extract being the maximum daily dosage considered for supplement purposes.

Blue Flag

Blue Flag has been used as a traditional supplement to help detoxify the body and alleviate the severity of acne, eczema, and psoriasis outbreaks.

Part Used:
Rhizome – Root

Side Effects:
Blue Flag is not recommended for use by women who are pregnant or nursing.

The fresh root of the blue flag may cause intestinal upset, nausea, and vomiting. The dried root has a milder effect.

Additional uses and side effects may exist but further research is necessary to determine the exact properties and effects of use.

General:
Blue Flag is native to the marshes of the United States where the Native Americans harvested the rhizome, dried and powdered it for use in internal and external traditional supplements.

Cleavers

Cleavers tea is traditionally used as part of an external wash or internal infusion treatment to detoxify the body and alleviate acne, eczema, and psoriasis.

Part Used:
Flower, Juice, Leaf

Side Effects:
Cleavers is not recommended for use by women who are pregnant or nursing.

Cleavers may affect blood sugar.

Cleavers is not recommended for use by people who are on blood thinning medication or who have a bleeding disorder.

Additional uses and side effects may exist but further research is necessary to determine the exact properties and effects of use.

General:
Cleavers is native to Africa, Asia, Europe, North America, and South America and has traditionally been harvested during the flowering season for use in a tea infusion made with 1 teaspoon of cleavers in 1 cup of hot water. Allow to steep. Use up to 3 times daily.

Coleus

Coleus contains enzymes that help to reduce inflammation that causes chronic skin conditions and is used in traditional treatments for eczema and psoriasis.

Part Used:
Root

Side Effects:
Coleus is not recommended for use by women who are pregnant or nursing.

Coleus has cardio-active effects and is not recommended for use without the advice of a physician or qualified herbalist.

Coleus is not recommended for use by people on asthma medication.

Coleus is not recommended for use by people who have hypotension. Coleus will lower the blood pressure.

Coleus is not recommended for use by people on blood thinning medication or who have a bleeding disorder.

Additional uses and side effects may exist but further research is necessary to determine the exact properties and effects of use.

General:
Coleus is native to Asia and India and cultivated elsewhere. Coleus root is often blended with other phyto-chemicals to aid in absorption since the root contains minute traces of each beneficial chemical. The therapeutic rate of Coleus Root is 50 milligrams 3 times daily.

Dandelion
Dandelion root helps the body to dispose of excess bacteria, toxins and hormones and has traditionally been used to help relieve skin conditions like acne, eczema, and psoriasis.

Part Used:
Leaf, Flower, Root

Side Effects:
Dandelion is not recommended for use by women who are pregnant or nursing.

Dandelion is not recommended for use by people with gall bladder disease without the guidance of a physician or qualified herbalist.

Dandelion is not recommended for use by people with stomach ulcers or gastritis.

Dandelion may cause stomach upset and diarrhea in some people.

Dandelion may cause an allergic reaction in some people.

General:
Dandelion is native to Asia, Europe, and North America where it is considered an invasive weed growing easily in a variety of sun, soil, and moisture conditions. It has been used by a variety of societies as a supplement treatment including the Native Americans. Dandelion leaf, flower, and root are used in salads, teas, and extracts and the flowers are sometimes used to make wine or in traditional teas up to 3 times daily.

Dulse

Dulse has been used as a traditional supplement to detoxify the body and alleviate certain skin conditions like acne, eczema, and psoriasis.

Part Used:
Leaf, Whole

Side Effects:
Dulse is not recommended for use by women who are pregnant or nursing.

Dulse is not recommended for use by people with hyperthyroidism.

Additional uses and side effects may exist but further research is necessary to determine the exact properties and effects of use.

General:
Dulse is a type of algae found on the coasts of both the Atlantic and Pacific oceans. It is harvested for use as a vegetable in some regions or for use in commercial supplements or traditional supplements.

Field Scabious

Field Scabious has traditionally been used as a tea tonic to promote faster healing and treat the symptoms of chronic or severe skin conditions like eczema, anal fissures, psoriasis, skin ulcers and wound care.

Part Used:
Flower, Leaf, Stem

Side Effects:
Field Scabious is not recommended for use by women who are pregnant or nursing.

Additional uses and side effects may exist but further research is necessary to determine the exact properties and effects of use.

General:
Field Scabious is found in nearly every region except the northernmost and southernmost parts of the world. It can be found growing in untended areas where the above ground parts are harvested, dried, and powdered for use in a traditional tea infusion.

Figwort

Figwort tea is traditionally used a detoxifier to reduce acne, eczema, and psoriasis outbreaks.

Part Used:
Flower, Leaf, Root, Stem

Side Effects:
Figwort is not recommended for use by women who are pregnant or nursing.

Figwort is not recommended for use by people with heart disease.

Figwort may affect blood sugar.

Additional uses and side effects may exist but further research is necessary to determine the exact properties and effects of use.

General:
Figwort is native to North America, Europe, and China where it is harvested before flowering for use as a tincture traditionally delivered at a rate of 15 drops up to 3 times a day.

Fumitory

Fumitory is used as a traditional supplement to detoxify the body and helps to clear skin conditions like acne, eczema, and psoriasis.

Part Used:
Flower, Leaf, Stem

Side Effects:
Fumitory is not recommended for use by women who are pregnant or nursing.

Overuse of Fumitory may cause diarrhea, trembling, convulsions and even death.

Additional uses and side effects may exist but further research is necessary to determine the exact properties and effects of use.

General:
Fumitory is native to Africa, Europe, and Siberia but has been naturalized to parts of North & South America where it is harvested for use as a grated, fresh supplement.

Sarsaparilla

Sarsaparilla has traditionally been used to detoxify the body and reduce impurity related flare-ups of conditions like acne, eczema, and psoriasis.

The phytochemicals in Sarsaparilla are believed to help sooth certain inflammatory conditions like acne, eczema, gout, and psoriasis by disabling certain bacterial components that build up in the blood and cause flare-ups in each condition.

Part Used:
Root

Side Effects:
Sarsaparilla is not recommended for use by women who are pregnant or nursing.

Sarsaparilla may cause asthma like symptoms in some people.

Over use or overdose of Sarsaparilla can cause kidney damage.

Additional uses and side effects may exist but further research is necessary to determine the exact properties and effects of use.

General:
Sarsaparilla is a woody climbing vine native to China, Central America & South America but cultivated in other regions. Sarsaparilla prefers rich, moist soil and part shade for optimal growth. Sarsaparilla is harvested in the late winter or early spring, dried and powdered for use in traditional supplements up to 3 times daily.

Appendix A - Skin Care Ingredients

Acacia - Gum
Acacia, Gum Arabic

Botanical Name:
Acacia senegal

Common Uses:
Binding Agents, Natural Skin Care

Traditional Uses:
Acacia Gum is often used as a stabilizer in creams and lotions and helps to improve the texture of semi-solid preparations.

Parts Used:
Gum

Side Effects:
Acacia is not recommended for use by women who are pregnant or nursing.

Acacia may cause an allergic reaction in some people.

Additional uses and side effects may exist but further research is necessary to determine the exact properties and effects of the root.

General:
Acacia is native to the semi-desert regions of Africa, Pakistan and India where the gum resin is harvested for use as a thickening agent or added to foods, cosmetic, or medicinal preparations.

Acacia Gum powder is soluble in water so it can be added to creams, lotions, liquid poultices, tooth care products, food products, and other items to stabilize the liquid and improve the texture of the final product.

1 tablespoon powdered gum to 3 tablespoons fluid creates a syrupy result.

Acacia Bark
Botanical Name:
Acacia decurrens

Common Uses:
Acne, Eczema, Natural Skin & Hair Care

Traditional Uses:
An herbal infusion of Acacia is believed to be a helpful component in anti-septic washes for the treatment of acne, eczema, and contact dermatitis.

Powdered Acacia is used as a binding agent for lotions, ointments and other semi-solids and is often used in natural skin care products.

Acacia bark is soluble in cold water.

Powdered Acacia Bark is added as a component in lotions to tighten skin and may help heal irritation.

Parts Used:
Bark - Powdered

Side Effects:
Acacia is not recommended for use by women who are pregnant or nursing.

Some people may have an allergic reaction to Acacia.

Overuse of Acacia can cause indigestion or constipation in some people.

Additional uses and side effects may exist but further research is necessary to determine the exact properties and effects.

General:
Acacia is native to the semi-desert regions of Africa, Pakistan and India. Acacia bark contains high levels of tannins and it is frequently used for tanning hides or is dried, and powdered for use in topical, culinary, and medicinal preparations.

1 tablespoon powdered bark to 3 tablespoons fluid creates a syrupy result.

Acacia, Umbrella Thorn
Botanical Name:
Acacia tortilis

Common Uses:
Skin Irritation, Thickening Agent

Traditional Use:
Powdered Umbrella Thorn bark is traditionally sprinkled over minor wounds and abrasions to aid in removing surface bacteria while maximizing the bodies healing ability.

Umbrella Thorn gum is used as a thickening alternative to Gum Arabic in many preparations.

Parts Used:
Bark, Leaf, Seed – Gum

Side Effects:
Acacia Umbrella Thorn is not recommended for use by women who are pregnant or nursing.

Umbrella Thorn may have a mild sedative effect and you should not drive or operate heavy machinery while using Umbrella Thorn.

Umbrella Thorn is recommended for topical use only.

Additional uses and side effects may exist but further research is necessary to determine the exact properties and effects.

General:
Umbrella Thorn is a canopied tree native to Africa that can also be found growing in the Middle East where it is harvested, dried, and powdered for use as a food product or in traditional supplement applications.

Agar
Botanical Name:
Gelidium amansii

Common Uses:
Natural Hair & Skin Care

Traditional Use:
Agar is a gelatin like thickening agent that shows a good balance between thickening and melting points making it a frequently used ingredient in cooking and natural product recipes.

Part Used:
Whole

Side Effects:
Agar is not recommended for use by women who are pregnant or nursing.

Agar is not recommended for individuals who have bowel obstruction.

Agar may result in poor absorption of nutrients and other medicines.

Agar must be taken with plenty of water.

If abdominal pain, chest pain, or difficulty swallowing occur you should see a physician or qualified herbalist immediately.

Additional uses and side effects may exist but further research is necessary to determine the exact properties and effects of use.

General:
Agar is a form of seaweed that is frequently used as a thickening agent in supplement, culinary, and cosmetic treatments. 1 teaspoon powder to 1 cup of boiling water creates a jelly like substance suitable for inclusion in a variety of recipes or traditionally delivered as 1 ounce of the gel up to 3 times daily with an adequate amount of fluids to be taken in addition to the gel.

Almond Oil
Botanical Name:
Prunus communis

Common Uses:
Contact Dermatitis, Natural Skin & Hair Care, Skin Irritation - Eczema, Carrier Oil

Traditional Use:
Almond oil is an easily absorbed oil with natural astringent & emollient actions making it useful in natural hair & skin care products.

Almond oil is used as a traditional skin lotion component to alleviate itchy skin conditions like contact dermatitis.

Almond is used in lotions and ointments to alleviate itchy skin conditions and promote a clear, younger looking complexion in any skin type.

Part Used:
Nut – Flour, Milk, Oil

Side Effects:
Almond oil should be extracted from the almond meat only.

Almond hull oils may be toxic in large quantities.

Additional uses and side effects may exist but further research is necessary to determine the exact properties and effects of use.

Aloe
Aloe, Aloe Vera, Burn Plant, Elephant's Gall, Lily of the Desert

Botanical Name:
Aloe Vera, Aloe barbadensis

Common Uses:
Acne, Contact Dermatitis, Natural Skin & Hair Care, Eczema, Psoriasis, Sun Burn Relief

Traditional Use:
Aloe is soothing, anti-inflammatory, and antibacterial making it a potentially beneficial ingredient for the treatment of acne.

Aloe gel is often used as a burn relief ointment. Most treatments thicken the juice with seaweed for easier application.

Aloe is sometimes used to treat minor skin wounds and abrasions. Aloe is believed speed wound healing by improving blood circulation and preventing cell death.

Aloe is emollient & believed to stimulate collagen regeneration making it a beneficial ingredient in natural skin and hair care products.

Aloe can be used in preparations to relieve the itchiness of eczema, poison ivy, ringworm, and psoriasis. It is typically created in an ointment using .5% aloe to a base.

Aloe is traditionally used as a poultice for wound care because it has antibacterial, antifungal, and antiviral compounds that help to prevent wound infections.

Part Used:
Gel, Juice, Leaf

Side Effects:
Aloe bitters and aloe juice should not be taken internally during pregnancy or menstruation or in cases of rectal bleeding.

The laxative compounds in aloe are passed into mother's milk, so nursing mothers should avoid internal use of aloe.

Aloe can cause intense intestinal cramps if overused.

Overuse of aloe juice can cause diarrhea.

The FDA banned the use of aloe as a laxative ingredient in over-the-counter drug products in 2002, but it is widely used outside the United States.

The oral consumption of aloe leaf may cause cancer.

Consumption of aloe may cause lowered glucose levels.

Additional uses and side effects may exist but further research is necessary to determine the exact properties and effects of use.

General:
Aloe is native to Africa but can be grown as a garden plant in other warm climates and is cultivated as an indoor plant worldwide. Aloe is related to the cactus and each part of the plant contains substances that are used in supplement treatments. The Aloe leaves contain a gel that is used as a topical ointment. The green part of the leaf that surrounds the gel is used to produce aloe juice or dried latex.

Aloe Butter is an extract of aloe in a coconut oil base. It is solid at room temperature but melts on the skin. It is traditionally incorporated into lotions & creams at a rate of 3-5%, in balms at a rate of 5-100%, and in conditioners at a rate of 2-5%.

Aloe Oil is used at a rate of 5-10% in recipes to add healing properties while lowering the risk of bacterial or mold growth.

Aloeswood
Agarwood, Aloeswood, Oudh

Botanical Name:

Aquilaria malaccensis

Common Uses:
Acne, Pigmentation, Skin Tonic

Traditional Use:
Aloeswood bark is traditionally used to help detoxify the body in the treatment of acne, gout, and rheumatism.

Aloeswood is traditionally used in skin tonic mixtures and may have pigment restoration qualities.

Powdered Aloeswood is traditionally sprinkled as an antiseptic on open wounds.

Part Used:
Wood, Bark – Powdered

Side Effects:
Additional uses and side effects may exist but further research is necessary to determine the exact properties and effects of use.

General:
Aloeswood comes from the Aquilaria Tree found growing naturally in Cambodia, India, and Vietnam and cultivated elsewhere. Aloeswood is commonly harvested, dried, and powdered for use as an incense, fabrication, and supplement products.

Andiroba Oil
Andiroba Oil, Bastard Mahogany, Carapa, Cedro, Crabwood

Botanical Name:
Carapa guianensis

Common Uses:
Age Spots, Eczema, Psoriasis, Skin Healing

Traditional Use:
Andiroba Oil contains mysteric acid that is believed to help minimize the growth of the pigment producing cells that cause age spots.

Andiroba oil contains myristic acid that tells skin cells when it is time to stop growing making it a potentially beneficial component in preventing the scales related to psoriasis and that plus the emollient properties make it a traditional component for the treatment of eczema.

Part Used:
Oil extracted from the nut, bark and leaves

Side Effects:
Andiroba Oil is for external use only.

Andiroba oil should not be used by women who are pregnant or nursing.

Additional uses and side effects may exist but further research is necessary to determine the exact properties and effects of use.

General:
Andiroba is native to the rainforests and is within the same family as mahogany making the wood valuable for many purposes. The oil is also extracted for supplement uses.

Angelica
Botanical Name:
Angelica archagelica

Common Uses:
Detoxification, Natural Skin Care, Psoriasis

Traditional Use:
Angelica oil is believed to be a detoxifier and is traditionally used to cleanse the blood and combat gout, psoriasis, and rheumatism.

Angelica oil is used in natural hair and skin care recipes and helps to brighten dull skin, remove toxins, and alleviate skin irritation.

Part Used:
Root, Seeds, Stalks

Side Effects:
Angelica is not for use by women who are pregnant or nursing. Angelica is a strong emmanagogue and can cause a miscarriage.

Angelica should be used with caution as large doses can negatively affect blood pressure, heart, and respiration. Angelica should only be considered for internal use after consultation with a physician or qualified herbalist.

Angelica fruits can cause sun sensitivity in some individuals.

Angelia oils can irritate the skin and mucus membranes.

Additional uses and side effects may exist but further research is necessary to determine the exact properties and effects of use.

General:
Angelica can be found growing in temperate zones along running streams & rivers. Angelica prefers dense shade and moist soil. Angelica is often supplied as a fluid extract at a rate of 1:1 with 1 teaspoon of the extract being the maximum daily dosage considered for supplement purposes.

Apple Vinegar
Apple Vinegar, Apple Cider Vinegar, Wine Vinegar

Botanical Name:

Malus domestica

Common Uses:
Natural Skin & Hair Care

Traditional Use:
Apple Vinegar has been used as a traditional skin wash to help speed healing in skin sores, ulcers, and wounds and to help remove warts.

Part Used:
Bark, Flowers, Fruit

Side Effects:
Apple seeds are toxic and should be consumed with caution.

Apple Cider Vinegar is not recommended for use beyond dietetic by women who are pregnant or nursing.

Apple Cider Vinegar may lower blood sugar.

Overuse of Apple Cider Vinegar may lower potassium.

Apple Cider Vinegar should be diluted before use.

Additional uses and side effects may exist for apple cider vinegar and whole books are available defining the believed properties and effects of use.

General:
The wild crab apple tree is now considered more beneficial than modernly cultivated apple trees.

Apples and Apple Vinegar are believed to have numerous uses and benefits. Entire books have been devoted to the uses of vinegar. The uses included here are believed to be the most commonly effective. You may wish to investigate a book specific to the uses and benefits of vinegar.

Apricot
Botanical Name:
Prunus armeniaca

Common Uses:
Contact Dermatitis, Eczema, Natural Skin &Hair Care, Skin Inflammation & Irritation

Carrier Oil

Traditional Use:
A decoction of the Apricot Bark is believed to be soothing to inflamed and irritated skin and is traditionally used to treat eczema and contact dermatitis.

Apricot Kernel oil is easily absorbed by the hair and skin making it a popular ingredient in natural skin & hair care recipes designed to infuse moisture without leaving a greasy feeling.

Apricot Kernel Oil is especially useful in moisturizing & nourishing aged, damaged, and sensitive skin.

Part Used:
Bark, Fruit, Seed - Oil

Side Effects:
Apricot is not recommended for use beyond dietary by women who are pregnant or nursing.

Apricot is generally considered safe when consumed as a food.

Apricot Kernel Oil is for external use only. Internal use of Apricot Kernel Oil is toxic.

Apricot may affect blood sugar and the dried fruit affects it more strongly than the fresh.

Additional uses and side effects may exist but further research is necessary to determine the exact properties and effects of use.

General:
Apricot is used as a food product by people around the world but it is also harvested for inclusion as a supplement and skin care ingredient. The apricot kernel is the seed of the fruit and is used to produce oils used for supplement purposes while the fruit itself is used in both topical and internal preparations.

Argan Oil
Botanical Name:
Argania spinosa

Common Uses:
Acne, Anti-Aging, Eczema, Healant, Natural Skin & Hair Care, Psoriasis

Traditional Use:
Argan Oil is rich in squalene and vitamins and is used to replace lost moisture while healing & protecting the skin. Argan oil has been used in traditional preparations to sooth skin ailments like acne, eczema, and psoriasis.

Argan Oil is rich in squalene and vitamins and is believed to replace lost moisture while limiting the effects of free radicals giving it a traditional use in anti-aging, smoothing, and strengthening products for the skin, hair, & nails.

Part Used:
Seed Oil

Side Effects:
Additional uses and side effects may exist but further research is necessary to determine the exact properties and effects of use.

General:

Argan Oil comes for the kernels of the Argan Tree native to Morocco and cultivation is being attempted elsewhere. Argan trees have been heavily commercialized and the oil has become very rare and costly. It is often combined with olive oil in treatments.

Arrowroot
Arrowroot, Maranta Starch

Botanical Name:
Maranta arundinacea

Common Uses:
Natural Hair & Skin Care, Thickening Agent

Traditional Use:
Arrowroot is used to thicken food, natural cosmetics, and supplement ointments, poultices, and creams.

Arrowroot has been used as a moist poultice to help draw poisons from bites & stings.

Part Used:
Root - Powdered

Side Effects:
Additional uses and side effects may exist but further research is necessary to determine the exact properties and effects of use.

General:
Arrowroot is native to Africa, Asia and Central America but has been naturalized to many warm regions where it is harvested, dried and powdered for use as a thickening agent in foods and cosmetics or as a traditional supplement.

Asphodelus
Botanical Name:
Asphodelus albus

Common Uses:
Natural Skin Care – Hyper-Pigmentation, Scarring

Traditional Use:
Asphodelus is used as part of a topical ointment or cream for fading freckles, age spots, scar tissue, and other undesirable skin pigmentation.

Part Used:
Tubers - Oil

Side Effects:
Additional uses and side effects may exist but further research is necessary to determine the exact properties and effects of use.

Asphodelus may cause skin irritation in some people.

General:

Asphodelus is a perennial native to Central and Southern Europe but is cultivated as an ornamental in other parts of the world. It is used in cheese making, ornamental gardens, and traditional supplements. The tubers are traditionally harvested in the spring, dried, and powdered for use in topical preparations.

Avens
Avens, Benedict's Herb, Bennet's Root, Benoite, Blessed Herb, Colewort, Geum, Herb Bennet

Botanical Name:
Geum urbanum

Common Uses:
Canker Sores, Hyper-Pigmentation,

Traditional Use:
Avens is traditionally used as a component in canker sore treatment sticks, ointments, and as a gargle for mouth sores.

Avens has been used as a wash to help to decrease the appearance of freckles, age spots and other hyper-pigmentation.

Part Used:
Flower, Leaf, Root, Stem

Side Effects:
Avens is not recommended for use by women who are pregnant or nursing.

Additional uses and side effects may exist but further research is necessary to determine the exact properties and effects of use.

General:
Avens is found in Asia, Europe, and North America where the root is harvested for use in external washes, poultices and traditional supplement teas or as a powder supplement.

Avocado
Alligator Pear, Avocado

Botanical Name:
Persea americana

Common Uses:
Dry & Damaged Skin, Eczema, Natural Skin and Hair Care, Psoriasis

Traditional Use:
Avocado and Avocado oil are rich in Vitamins B, E, and K making them a key ingredient in many deep moisture skin masks, deep skin treatments, and hair treatments. Avocado is especially beneficial for mature or damaged skin as it helps to hydrate and nourish regenerating skin cells. Avocado is not recommended for oily skin and is frequently used for its ability to screen harmful sun rays.

Avocado oil may help to reduce the symptoms of extremely dry skin, eczema, and psoriasis when ingested as part of a supplement diet or applied as a topical ointment.

Part Used:
Fruit, Oil, Seed

Side Effects:
Avocado is not recommended for use beyond dietary by women who are pregnant or nursing.

Avocado may cause an allergic reaction in some people.

Additional uses and side effects may exist but further research is necessary to determine the exact properties and effects of use.

General:
Avocados are native to subtropical regions and do not tolerate frost. If you cultivate avocado indoors, you must have multiple trees to promote cross-pollination. To start a sprout pierce a seed from a ripe avocado 3 or 4 times and place it in a glass of water. Avocado is used as a food in many cultures and is a good source of potassium and Vitamin D. Avocado is also harvested for use in traditional supplements and dietary treatments.

Balloon Vine
Botanical Name:
Cardiospermum halicacabum

Common Uses:
Acne, Contact Dermatitis, Eczema

Traditional Use:
Dried Balloon Vine leaves are traditionally boiled into a tea at a rate of 2 tablespoons to 1-cup water that is used internally to reduce acne, eczema, and other skin conditions.

A poultice of balloon vine leaves can be applied as a hot poultice for relief from the pain and swelling associated with arthritis, joint injury, muscle pain and other painful inflammatory conditions.

Balloon Vine leaves have been used in traditional topical ointments to help alleviate the pain & inflammation and speed healing in wounds and ulcers.

Part Used:
Leaves, Seeds, Vine - Whole

Side Effects:
Balloon Vine is not recommended for use by women who are pregnant or nursing.

Additional uses and side effects may exist but further

research is necessary to determine the exact properties and effects of use.

General:
Balloon Vine is a perennial native to Central and South America and cultivated by seed as a climbing vine where it is harvested for use fresh or dried in traditional supplement preparations.

Bamboo Brier
Bamboo Brier, Greenbriar

Botanical Name:
Smilax rotundifolia

Common Uses:
Eczema, Contact Dermatitis, Thickening Agent

Traditional Use:
The stem and prickles of bamboo brier can be rubbed on skin to lessen the effect of environmental irritants, contact dermatitis, and eczema.

The root of the bamboo brier is boiled or dried and powdered for use as a thickening agent in foods, cosmetics, and supplements.

Part Used:
Leaf, Prickle, Root, Stem

Side Effects:
Bamboo Brier is not recommended for use by women who are pregnant or nursing.

Bamboo Brier may cause an allergic reaction or skin irritation in some people.
Additional uses and side effects may exist but further research is necessary to determine the exact properties and effects of use.

General:
Bamboo Brier is a woody vine native to the United States where it can be found growing wild along roadsides and woodland clearings. The shoots are harvested for use as a food eaten fresh in salads or cooked like asparagus and the roots are boiled or powdered for use as a thickening agent.

Baobab
Adansonia, Boabab, Cream of Tarter Tree, Boki, Senegal, Upside Down Tree

Botanical Name:
Adansonia digitata

Common Uses:
Anti-Aging, Carrier Oil, Contact Dermatitis, Eczema, Natural Hair & Skin Care, Psoriasis

Traditional Use:
Baobab oil is rich in nutrients, helps to improve skin elasticity, regenerate cells, and does not clog pores

making it prized in natural skin care products especially those designed to treat aged or damaged skin.

Baobab oil is traditionally used in ointments and washes to minimize the inflammation and itching associated with contact dermatitis, eczema and psoriasis.

Baobab oil is a highly moisturizing emollient that soothes the skin while rejuvenating the cells making it a prized component in natural hair & skin care products.

Part Used:
Bark, Fruit, Leaf, Seed - Oil

Side Effects:
Baobab is not recommended for use by women who are pregnant or nursing.

Additional uses and side effects may exist but further research is necessary to determine the exact properties and effects of use.

General:
The Baobab is a tree native to Africa and naturalized to most tropical countries where it is harvested as a food for the indigenous peoples. Baobab has a unique nutritional content and is considered by some to be the next likely super food. Baobab oils are extracted by cold pressing the seeds and the bark and leaves are harvested, dried, and powdered for use in traditional supplement preparations.

Basil
Albahaca, Basil, Garden Basil, Munjariki, Surasa, Varvara

Botanical Name:
Ocimum basilicum

Common Uses:
Acne, Natural Hair & Skin Care

Traditional Use:
Basil is traditionally included in skin washes to tone and brighten the skin and may be beneficial in treating certain types of bacterial acne.

Side Effects:
Basil is not recommended for use beyond dietary by women who are pregnant or nursing

Basil is not recommended for use beyond dietary in children's treatment.

Basil is not for long-term use.

Additional uses and side effects may exist but further research is necessary to determine the exact properties and effects of use.

General:

Basil is a commonly cultivated spice herb that grows easily from seed, Basil prefers full sunlight, fertile soil, and steady moisture and is often used as a seasoning or dried for use as a supplement tea.

Bay
Bay, Bay Laurel, Daphne, Grecian Laurel, Mediterranean Bay, Roman Laurel, Sweet Bay, True Bay

Botanical Name:
Laurus nobilis

Common Uses:
Natural Skin Care

Traditional Use:
Bay leaves added to a pot of boiling water for use as a deep cleansing steam treatment for the face.

Part Used:
Fruit, Leaves, Oil

Side Effects:
Bay is not recommended for use beyond dietary by women who are pregnant or nursing.

Bay may cause an allergic reaction in some people.

Bay may irritate the skin and mucus membranes of some individuals and should be used with caution

Bay oil should not be taken internally. Oil is for external use only.

Additional uses and side effects may exist but further research is necessary to determine the exact properties and effects of use.

General:
Bay Laurel is not a winter hardy plant and should be brought indoors in much of the northern parts of the country. Bay prefers full sun light and good drainage.

Bayberry – Sweet Gale
Bayberry, Bog Myrtle, Dutch Myrtle, Sweet Gale

Botanical Name:
Myrica gale

Common Uses:
Acne, Natural Skin Care – Redness, Seborrhea

Traditional Use:
Sweet Gale has been used in traditional topical washes and spot ointments to alleviate the severity of acne outbreaks and some types of skin redness including seborrhea.

Sweet Gale is used in natural skin care preparations to help reduce acne, inflammation redness, and seborrhea.

Part Used:
Branch, Leaf, Wax

Side Effects:
Sweet Gale is not recommended for use by women who are pregnant or nursing.

Sweet Gale has been used as an abortifacient in some cultures.

Additional uses and side effects may exist but further research is necessary to determine the exact properties and effects of use.

General:
Sweet Gale is a deciduous shrub native to Europe and North America where it is cultivated as an ornamental or harvested for use in topical preparations and as a flavoring.

Bear's Breeches
Botanical Name:
Acanthus mollis

Common Uses:
Contact Dermatitis

Traditional Use:
Bear's Breeches are incorporated into traditional topical preparations to sooth skin irritation associated with contact dermatitis and speed wound healing.

Part Used:
Flower, Leaf

Side Effects:
Bear's Breeches are not recommended for use by women who are pregnant or nursing.

Bear's Breeches may cause an allergic reaction in some people.

Additional uses and side effects may exist but further research is necessary to determine the exact properties and effects of use.

General:
Bear's Breeches is native to Europe but has been naturalized to Asia and North America where it can be found growing wild in damp areas or cultivated as a ground cover where it is harvested for use in traditional supplements.

Beech
Beech, Boke, Faggio

Botanical Name:
Fagus grandifolia

Common Uses:
Contact Dermatitis

Traditional Use:
The fresh or dried beech leaves are traditionally used as a poultice to sooth burns.

A tea made of the fresh bark has traditionally been used as a topical wash to help alleviate skin rashes, itchiness, and speed healing in poison ivy and other forms of eruptive contact rashes.

Part Used:
Bark, Leaf, Oil, Resin

Side Effects:
Beech is not recommended for use by women who are pregnant or nursing.

Beech may cause an allergic reaction or skin irritation in some people.

Additional uses and side effects may exist but further research is necessary to determine the exact properties and effects of use.

General:
The Beech is native to Europe and North America where the nut is forage for animals and occasionally eaten by people, the oils are used in supplements, and the resin is harvested, dried, and powdered for use in traditional supplements.

Benzoin
Benjamin Tree, Benjoin, Benzoe, Benzoin Resin, Friar's Balsam, Lohban

Botanical Name:
Styrax benzoin

Common Uses:
Eczema

Traditional Use:
Benzoin resin is used in many commercial skin protective products and has been used in traditional supplements to heal chapped or blistered skin and to relieve skin blisters, irritation, sores, and ulcers.

Benzoin is often included in washes to help speed the healing of inflamed, irritated, or cracked skin especially in conditions such as eczema.

Part Used:
Bark Resin

Side Effects:
Benzoin is not recommended for use by women who are pregnant or nursing.

Excessive amounts of Benzoin can cause drowsiness.

Additional uses and side effects may exist but further research is necessary to determine the exact properties and effects of use.

General:
The Benzoin Tree is native to Sumatra where the tree is wounded to cause resin production. The resin is then harvested for use in supplement preparations perfumes, and incense.

Bergamot
Beebalm, Bergamot, Fragrant Balm, High Balm, Indian Plume, Mountain Balm

Botanical Name:
Bergamot didyma, Citrus bergamia

Common Uses:
Acne

Traditional Use:
Bergamot is an antibacterial, antiviral, analgesic and may be beneficial in treatments for certain types of acne when added to topical preparations at a rate of 1 to 10.

Part Used:
Fruit, Leaf, Peel Oil

Side Effects:
Bergamot is not recommended for use by women who are pregnant or nursing.

Bergamot is not recommended for use in children's treatments.

Bergamot increases sun sensitivity. Do not use on the skin when sun exposure is likely.

Additional uses and side effects may exist but further research is necessary to determine the exact properties and effects of use.

General:
Bergamot is native to Asia and can grow up to 16 feet in height. Bergamot is harvested for use in topical & internal preparations as well as in fragrances, inhalant therapy, and natural care products.

Bitter Damson
Bitter Damson, Dysentery Bark, Mountain Damson, Simarouba, Slave Wood, Stave Wood

Botanical Name:
Simarouba amara

Common Uses:
Hyper-Pigmentation, Natural Skin Care

Traditional Uses:
Bitter Damson has been used in commercial and traditional topical preparations to fade freckles, age

spots, and scarring and is valued as a natural skin care ingredient for its hydrating effect.

Parts Used:
Bark

Side Effects:
Bitter Damson is not for use by women who are pregnant or nursing.

Bitter Damson has been used as an abortifacient. Overuse of Bitter Damson may cause gastrointestinal upset.

Additional uses and side effects may exist but further research is necessary to determine the exact properties and effects of use.

General:
Bitter Damson is native to the Caribbean and South America where the bark is harvested, dried, and powdered for use in traditional supplement. Bitter Damson has recently gained interest by researches for its potential in treating viral infections, stimulating the immune system, and preventing or treating cancer.

Bittersweet - American
American Bittersweet, False Bittersweet, Waxwork

Botanical Name:
Celastrus scandens

Common Uses:
Contact Dermatitis, Skin Irritation

Traditional Use:
American Bittersweet is traditionally used in washes, ointments, and poultices to help speed healing in burns, contact dermatitis, and minor skin irritation.

Part Used:
Root Bark

Side Effects:
American Bittersweet is not recommended for use by women who are pregnant or nursing.

Additional uses and side effects may exist but further research is necessary to determine the exact properties and effects of use.

General:
American bittersweet is a shrub native to North America and can be found growing wild in thickets throughout the northern portion of the country where the root bark is harvested, dried and powdered for use in traditional supplement infusions.

Black Catechu
Black Catechu, Black Cutch, Cachou, Cutch, Gambier

Botanical Name:

Acacia catechu

Common Uses:
Acne, Contact Dermatitis, Eczema

Traditional Use:
Black Catechu has traditionally been incorporated into a wash for the treatment of acne, eczema, and other eruptive skin conditions.

Part Used:
Bark, Heartwood, Leaf

Side Effects:
Black Catchu is not recommended for use by women who are pregnant or nursing.

Black Catechu may lower blood pressure.

Additional uses and side effects may exist but further research is necessary to determine the exact properties and effects of use.

General:
Black Catechu is native to India where the bark is boiled to extract the dye properties or harvested, dried and powdered for use as a breath freshener, diuretic, colorant or traditional supplement.

Black Currant
Black Currant, Cassis

Botanical Name:
Ribes nigrum

Common Uses:
Natural Skin Care

Traditional Uses:
Blackcurrant oil is sometimes used as a replacement for evening primrose oil in natural skin care recipes.

Black Current has been used as a traditional wash to help speed the healing of minor wounds and skin ulcers.

Parts Used:
Fruit, Leaf, Seed – Oil

Side Effects:
Black Currant is not recommended for use by women who are pregnant or nursing.

Black current might slow blood clotting.

Additional uses and side effects may exist but further research is necessary to determine the exact properties and effects of use.

General:
Black Current is a berry native to Asia, Europe and cultivated elsewhere. The fruit is harvested as a food or

drink component and for use as a dietary supplement. The leaves are harvested for use fresh or dried in traditional topical and tea supplements.

Black Jujube
Azufaifo, Badar, Ber, Black Date, Black Jujube, Chinese Date, Da Zao, Jujube Plum, Red Date

Botanical Name:
Ziziphus jujuba

Common Uses:
Natural Skin Care

Traditional Uses:
Jujube extracts are used in commercial and natural products to help reduce redness in the skin while combating wrinkles and premature aging.

Parts Used:
Fruit

Side Effects:
Jujube is not recommended for use by women who are pregnant or nursing.

Jujube is not recommended for use by people who are trying to conceive.

Jujube may lower the blood pressure.

Additional uses and side effects may exist but further research is necessary to determine the exact properties and effects of use.

General:
Black Jujube is a shrub or tree native to Asia and Europe. The fruit is harvested for use as a food product and for use in traditional supplements.

Black Spruce
Botanical Name:
Picea mariana, Pinus nigra

Common Uses:
Skin Wounds – Contact Dermatitis, Thickening Agent

Traditional Use:
The resin of the black spruce is harvested for use as a gummy agent in supplement and personal product creation.

The bark of the Black Spruce is sometimes used as a thickening agent in both culinary and supplement treatments especially topical preparations designed to sooth inflamed and irritated skin.

Part Used:
Bark

Side Effects:

Black Spruce is not recommended for use by women who are pregnant or nursing.

Black Spruce may cause an allergic reaction in some people.

Additional uses and side effects may exist but further research is necessary to determine the exact properties and effects of use.

General:
The Black Spruce is native to North America where the bark is harvested, dried and powdered for use in traditional supplement treatments. The gum resin, cones, and branches are harvested for use as colorants, food products, and personal care products.

Blackthorn
Black Thorn, Blackthorn, Sloe, Wild Plum

Botanical Name:
Prunus spinosa

Common Uses:
Acne, Skin Inflammation

Traditional Uses:
Blackthorn flowers have been used in traditional topical preparations to deep cleanse the skin and alleviate certain types of acne.

Blackthorn flower is traditionally added to a poultice or wash to help sooth inflamed and irritated skin.

Parts Used:
Berry, Flower

Side Effects:
Black Thorn is not recommended for use by women who are pregnant or nursing.

Black Thorn may cause an allergic reaction in some people.

Additional uses and side effects may exist but further research is necessary to determine the exact properties and effects of use.

General:
Black Thorn is a deciduous shrub native to Africa, Asia, Europe and North America where it is cultivated as a naturally barbed hedge. The fruit is harvested as a jam or wine component and the fruit, flowers, and leaves are used in traditional supplements.

Boneset
Agueweed, Boneset, Crosswort, Feverwort, Indian Sage, Sweating Plant, Teasel, Thoroughwort, Wood Boneset

Botanical Name:
Eupatorium perfoliatum

Common Uses:
Acne, Contact Dermatitis, Eczema

Traditional Use:
Boneset has been used in traditional topical preparations to alleviate the symptoms of acne, eczema, and contact dermatitis.

Part Used:
Whole – After Flowering

Side Effects:
Boneset is not recommended for use by women who are pregnant or nursing.

Boneset is an immuno-stimulant and is not recommended for use by people who have an immune sensitive disorder like Multiple Sclerosis or Lupus.

Boneset may cause allergic reactions in those who suffer from seasonal allergies related to chamomile, ragwort, and others.

Overdose of Boneset may cause diarrhea, nausea, and vomiting.

Additional uses and side effects may exist but further research is necessary to determine the exact properties and effects of use.

General:
Boneset is native to the United States where it can be found growing wild in moist areas like swamp edges and stream banks. The entire herb is harvested after flowering and made into a traditional supplement tea up to 3 times daily or tincture traditionally given as ¾ teaspoon before meals.

Borage
Bee Plant, Beebread, Borage, Borago, Borraja, Cool Tankard, Ox's Tongue, Talewort, Starflower

Botanical Name:
Borago officinalis

Common Uses:
Eczema, Mature Body Lotion, Skin Restoration, Sun Damage

Traditional Use:
Borage seed oil contains higher levels of GLA than nearly any other plant source and has proven beneficial in topical and internal treatments for aged skin, eczema, psoriasis, and other skin disorders. Borage oils are mixed with other oils at a rate of 10% and have a regenerating and stimulating effect for all skin types.

Part Used:
Flower, Leaves, Seed Oils

Side Effects:
Borage is not recommended for use by women who are pregnant or nursing.

Borage is not recommended for use by people who have a bleeding disorder, are undergoing surgery, or who have a liver condition.

Borage is not recommended for long term use.

Borage Seed Oil contains amounts of pyrrolizidine alkaloids that may damage the liver, cause cancer, or other conditions. Only PA Free Borage is used in traditional supplement.

Additional uses and side effects may exist but further research is necessary to determine the exact properties and effects of use.

General:
Borage requires well drained, acidic soil with moderate to high levels of sunlight. Borage grows to approximately 12 inches in width and will spread easily. The flowers & leaves are harvested for use in traditional supplement infusions and the oil is extracted from the seed for use in other preparations.

Brown Kelp
Alginate, Brown Kelp, Pacific Kelp, Sea Kelp, Sea Whistle

Botanical Name:
Macrocystis pyrifera

Common Uses:
Natural Hair & Skin Care

Traditional Use:
Brown Kelp is used as a binding agent in supplement and natural care products and is sometimes used as a peel off facial masks.

Part Used:
Whole

Side Effects:
Brown kelp is not recommended for use by women who are pregnant or nursing.

Brown kelp is a source of iodine and should not be used by those who have hyperthyroidism.

Additional uses and side effects may exist but further research is necessary to determine the exact properties and effects of use.

General:
Brown kelp is found primarily along the California coastline and is harvested for use as a binding agent and in traditional supplements.

Caje Oil

Caje Oil, Huile, Niauli

Botanical Name:
Melaleuca viridiflora

Common Uses:
Acne, Skin Inflammation

Concentration, Focus

Traditional Uses:
Caje Oil has been used in traditional topical preparations to clean oily skin and combat bacteria in certain types of acne and to prevent infection and speed healing in skin ulcers and wounds.

Caje oil is applied directly to the throat, mouth, or skin to reduce inflammation and is traditionally believed to be most effective at treating bacterial infections and associated inflammation.

Parts Used:
Leaf, Twigs - Oil

Side Effects:
Caje Oil is not recommended for use by women who are pregnant or nursing.

Caje Oil is not recommended for use in children's treatments.

Caje Oil may cause diarrhea, nausea or vomiting.

Overuse of Caje Oil may cause breathing problems, circulation problems, and low blood pressure.

Additional uses and side effects may exist but further research is necessary to determine the exact properties and effects of use.

General:
Caje Oil is extracted from the leaves of the Melaleuca viridiflora plant and should not be confused with cajeput oil that is taken from a different species of the Melaleuca plant. The Melaleuca viridiflora is native to Australia where the bark is used as bedding, containers, and building shelter. The essential oil is extracted from young leaves and twigs for use in traditional supplement and disinfectant preparations.

Cajeput
Cajeput, Paperbark Tree, Swamp Tea Tree, White Tea Tree

Botanical Name:
Melaleuca leucadendron

Common Uses:
Acne, Eczema, Psoriasis

Traditional Use:

Cajeput oil has been used as part of a topical wash or ointment preparation to help alleviate the severity of acne, eczema and psoriasis outbreaks.

Part Used:
Leaves, Twigs

Side Effects:
Cajeput is not recommended for use by women who are pregnant or nursing.

Cajeput is not recommended in children's treatments.

Cajeput is not recommended for use by people with kidney problems.

Cajeput may worsen asthma symptoms in some people.

Cajeput may cause skin irritation. You should dilute it before applying cajeput to the skin and it is not recommended for use in the facial area.

Additional uses and side effects may exist but further research is necessary to determine the exact properties and effects of use.

General:
Cajeput is native to Australia and Asia preferring extremely wet conditions for optimal growth. Cajeput oil is extracted from the leaves and twigs of the tree and blended with other oils for use as a traditional supplement diluted at 5 drops cajeput to 1 tablespoon carrier oil.

Calendula
Bull Flower, Calendula, Gold Bloom, Holligold, Marigold, Mercadela, Pot Marigold, Zergul

Botanical Name:
Calendula officinalis

Common Uses:
Acne, Natural Skin Care

Traditional Use:
Calendula blossoms are anti-inflammatory, astringent, and anti-bacterial making them a traditional component in topical ointments for acne, burns, bruises, and minor wounds. Simmer with preferred ingredients and apply directly to the skin or include in a lotion recipe.

Calendula is traditionally used to cleanse and accelerate healing in minor wounds, bed sores, and ulcers.

Part Used:
Flowers, Oil

Side Effects:

Calendula is not recommended for use by women who are pregnant or nursing.

Calendula has been used as a male contraceptive and should not be used by men and women who are trying to conceive.

Calendula may cause an allergic reaction in some people.

Additional uses and side effects may exist but further research is necessary to determine the exact properties and effects of use.

General:
Calendula is native to the Mediterranean but is cultivated as an annual garden plant in much of the world. It is easy to grow from seed and should be harvested while in bloom. Calendula is traditionally dried and powdered for use as a tea up to 3 times daily but has also been used as a tincture or topical salve additive.

Camphor
Botanical Name:
Cinnamomum camphora

Common Uses:
Acne, Contact Dermatitis, Eczema, Natural Hair & Skin Care, Skin Irritation

Traditional Use:
Camphor oil is traditionally used in topical preparations to combat oily skin and acne.

Camphor has been approved for use in Europe as a topical cream to reduce skin itching and irritation from contact dermatitis, excessive dryness, and for conditions like eczema.

Part Used:
Wood – Steam Distilled Oils

Side Effects:
Camphor is not recommended for use by women who are pregnant or nursing.

Camphor is not recommended for topical applications in children.

Camphor may irritate skin and should not be applied to broken skin or large areas.

Use only cosmetic grade white camphor.

Camphor is for external use only.

Additional uses and side effects may exist but further research is necessary to determine the exact properties and effects of use.

General:

True Cinnamomum camphora is the waxy white substance extracted from the Camphor Laurel Tree native to Asia but camphor can be found in the bark of a variety of trees in smaller amounts than the Cinnamomum camphora. The bark is harvested and the oils extracted for use at a rate of up to 10% in traditional supplement preparations.

Carline Thistle
Carlina, Carline Thistle, Dwarf Carline, Ground Thistle, Stemless Carline

Botanical Name:
Carlina acaulis

Common Uses:
Acne, Contact Dermatitis, Eczema

Traditional Use:
Carline Thistle oils are traditionally included in a skin wash to alleviate the symptoms of acne, contact dermatitis, eczema, and skin ulcers and are believed to speed the healing process.

Carline Thistle is traditionally included in topical washes and ointments to prevent infection and speed healing of skin sores, ulcers and wounds.

Part Used:
Root - Oil

Side Effects:
Carline Thistle is not recommended for use by women who are pregnant or nursing.

Carline Thistle may cause an allergic reaction in some people.

Additional uses and side effects may exist but further research is necessary to determine the exact properties and effects of use.

General:
Carline Thistle is found in many areas of Europe and the United States where the root is harvested in the fall and dried for use in tea traditionally given at a rate of 2 teaspoons root powder to 1 cup of water 3 times daily or steam distilled to extract the essential oils.

Carob
Algarrobo, Carob, Garrofero, Locust Bean, St. John's Bread, Sugar Pods

Botanical Name:
Ceratonia siliqua

Common Uses:
Natural Skin Care

Traditional Use:
Carob is included in natural skin care products to help to cleanse the face and tone the skin.

Part Used:
Bark, Seed

Side Effects:
Carob is not recommended for use beyond dietary by women who are pregnant or nursing.

Do not take Vitamin A supplements when using carob supplements.

Carob may increase the effects of digoxin in some individuals.

Additional uses and side effects may exist but further research is necessary to determine the exact properties and effects of use.

General:
Carob is native to Asia, Europe and the Mediterranean but it has been cultivated in North America. Carob is often used as a dietary additive by dissolving the powder in an equal part of cold liquid. Boil for 1 minute to create a thickening agent.

Carrot
Beesnest Plant, Bird's Nest Root, Carrot, Wild Carrot, Queen Anne's Lace

Botanical Name:
Daucus carota

Common Uses:
Natural Skin Care

Traditional Use:
Carrot seed oil helps to balance the oils in the skin, heal damage, and may be beneficial in aged skin care.

Part Used:
Leaf, Seed

Side Effects:
Carrot is not recommended for use by women who are pregnant or nursing.

Carrot Seed is a natural abortifacient.

Carrot Seed had been used as a morning after contraceptive in some cultures and is not recommended for use by women trying to conceive.

Wild Carrot may cause an allergic reaction in some people.

Wild Carrot may affect the kidneys.

Additional uses and side effects may exist but further research is necessary to determine the exact properties and effects of use.

General:

Wild carrot is native to Eastern North America, Europe, and Asia. It is often found growing in untended fields and along roadsides where it is harvested and juiced or made into a traditional supplement syrup.

Castor
African Coffee Tree, Castor Bean, Castor bean, Castor Oil, Reanda, Mexico Weed, Ricine, Tangantangan Oil, Wonder Tree

Botanical Name:
Ricinus communis

Common Uses:
Natural Skin Care

Traditional Use:
Castor oil is a hard, shiny oil that can be used to protect the skin from the elements and is used in lotions for extreme weather conditions.

Part Used:
Seed Oil

Side Effects:
The hull of the castor seed is poisonous.

Castor is not recommended for use by women who are pregnant or nursing.

Castor oil has abortifacient properties.

Castor is not recommended for women who are trying to conceive, as it is believed to be a long-term contraceptive.

Castor is not recommended for use in children's treatments.

Castor Oil may cause cramping and nausea.

Additional uses and side effects may exist but further research is necessary to determine the exact properties and effects of use.

General:
Castor plants are native to the Middle East and Africa but are cultivated in many tropical regions where the seeds are harvested and the oils extracted for use in commercial and traditional preparations.

Centaury
Bitter Herb, Centaury, Feverwort

Botanical Name:
Centaurium erythraea

Common Uses:
Hyper-Pigmentation, Natural Skin Care

Traditional Use:

An infusion of Centaury may help to clear blemishes, soften the skin and remove dark pigmentation so it is often used in natural skin care.

Part Used:
Flower, Leaf

Side Effects:
Centaury is not recommended for use by women who are pregnant or nursing.

Centaury should not be used with stomach or intestinal ulcers.

Additional uses and side effects may exist but further research is necessary to determine the exact properties and effects of use.

General:
Centaury is native to Asia, Africa and Europe and cultivated in the United States where it is harvested during the flowering season and dried quickly for use as a traditional tea supplement.

Chamomile - German
Blue Chamomile, German Chamomile, Hungarian Chamomile, Kamillen, Kleine Kamille, Manzanilla, Matricaire Camomille. Pin Heads, Sweet False Chamomile, True Chamomile, Wild Chamomile

Botanical Name:
Chamomilla recutita, Matricaria recutita

Common Uses:
Eczema, Natural Face, Hair & Skin Care

Traditional Use:
A poultice of strong chamomile tea can be applied to relieve the appearance of tired, puffy eyes.

Chamomile is used in natural hair, skin, & face care treatments.

Part Used:
Flowers

Side Effects:
Chamomile may not be recommended for use by women who are pregnant or nursing.

Chamomile is not recommended for use by women who have a hormone sensitive condition like endometriosis, fibroids, or certain types of cancer.

Chamomile is not recommended for use by people who are taking prescription blood thinners or suffering from a disorder where blood thinners are counter indicated.

Chamomile may cause an allergic reaction such as skin rashes, throat swelling, and shortness of breath in those who are allergic to plants in the ragweed family.

Additional uses and side effects may exist but further research is necessary to determine the exact properties and effects of use.

General:
Chamomile is native to Europe but has been naturalized as a landscape and herb plant in much of the word. Chamomile is easy to grow from seed. The flowering tops of the chamomile plant are used in tea, extract, and capsule form and can be applied whole to sooth skin conditions or chewed for mouth conditions. 2 tsp to 1 cup hot water, steep 30 minutes. Up to 3 cups per day

The flowers of another species of chamomile Anthemis tinctoria known as dyer's chamomile yield a yellow toned colorant. Mordant – Alum

Chaparral
Chaparral, Creosote Bush, Greasewood, Hedionilla, Jarilla

Botanical Name:
Larrea tridentata

Common Uses:
Acne, Natural Skin Care – Burns, Eczema, Psoriasis

Traditional Use:
Chaparral tincture is used as a traditional ingredient in short term alcohol based topical treatments for acne, burns, contact dermatitis, eczema, and psoriasis

Part Used:
Flower, Leaf, Fruit

Side Effects:
Chaparral is not recommended for use by women who are pregnant or nursing.

Chaparral is for external use only – prolonged ingestion of chaparral can cause liver damage.

Chaparral is not recommended for long term use.

Chaparral may cause diarrhea, fever, headache, kidney damage, liver damage, nausea, stomach pain, weight loss, and allergic skin reactions.

Additional uses and side effects may exist but further research is necessary to determine the exact properties and effects of use.

General:
Chaparral is native to the Southwestern regions of the United States and Mexico where it is harvested for use as a tincture or traditional supplement up to 3 times daily.

Chervil
Chervil, Sweet Cicely

Botanical Name:
Anthriscus cerfolium

Common Uses:
Contact Dermatitis

Traditional Use:
Chervil tea has traditionally been used as a skin wash, ointment, or poultice to alleviate the discomfort associated with bites, stings, and eruptive contact dermatitis.

Part Used:
Juice, Seed, Whole Herb

Side Effects:
Chervil is not recommended for use by women who are pregnant or nursing.

Additional uses and side effects may exist but further research is necessary to determine the exact properties and effects of use.

General:
Chervil is native to Russia and Asia but has been cultivated worldwide as a pot or kitchen herb. Chervil grows easily from seeds and prefers rich soil with good drainage and full sun. It is harvested as a culinary seasoning and used in traditional supplement salves and infusions.

Chickweed
Adder's Mouth, Chickweed, Star Chickweed, Starweed

Botanical Name:
Stellaria media

Common Uses:
Acne, Contact Dermatitis, Eczema, Psoriasis, Seborrhea

Traditional Use:
Chickweed is used as part of a cooling, anti-inflammatory ointment for conditions such as acne, eczema, hemorrhoids, and psoriasis.

Chickweed has been used in traditional topical ointment or poultice preparations to reduce the appearance of redness of the skin in conditions like seborrhea.

Part Used:
Flower, Leaf, Root, Stem

Side Effects:
Chickweed is cultivated as a kitchen herb and is generally considered safe for consumption.

Chickweed is not recommended for use beyond dietary by women who are pregnant or nursing.

Chickweed may cause diarrhea.

Chickweed may cause an allergic reaction or skin irritation in some people.

Additional uses and side effects may exist but further research is necessary to determine the exact properties and effects of use.

General:
Chickweed is native to Asia and Europe but has naturalized throughout much the world and is considered a weed by some. The leaves have been used as a cold vegetable and the whole plant has been used in traditional supplements treat a variety of ailments in tea and poultice applications.

Chlorophyll
Botanical Name:
Chlorophyll

Common Uses:
Natural Skin Care – Acne, Healing, Wound Care

Traditional Use:
Chlorophyll has been used in traditional topical preparations to speed wound healing.

Chlorophyll has traditionally been used to cleanse the body, oxygenate blood, and encourage new cell growth.

Chlorophyll has been used as a component in natural skin care products designed to promote healing and maintain healthy, blemish free skin.

Part Used:
Extract

Side Effects:
Chlorophyll is not recommended for use by women who are pregnant or nursing.

Overuse of chlorophyll may cause abdominal cramps, diarrhea, or gastrointestinal upset.

Chlorophyll is not recommended for use without the advice of a physician or qualified herbalist.

Additional uses and side effects may exist but further research is necessary to determine the exact properties and effects of use.

General:
Chlorophyll is the green pigment found in plants and algae. Chlorophyll is extracted from the plant and used as a dietary supplement, cosmetic, and traditional liquid supplement.

Clary Sage
Clary Sage, Clary Wort, Clear Eye, Eyebright, Muscatel Sage, See Bright

Botanical Name:
Salvia sclarea

Common Uses:
Natural Skin and Hair Care

Traditional:
Clary sage is an excellent treatment for oily hair and skin and for dandruff control treatments.

Part Used:
Flower, Leaf

Side Effects:
Clary Sage is not recommended for use by women who are pregnant or nursing.

Clary Sage is not recommended for use by women who have a hormone sensitive condition like endometriosis, fibroids or certain types of cancer.

Additional uses and side effects may exist but further research is necessary to determine the exact properties and effects of use.

General:
Clary Sage is native to Italy and Syria but is cultivated worldwide as a culinary additive, perfume, aromatherapy treatment and traditional supplement.

Club Moss
Chinese Club Moss, Club Moss, Stag's Horn, Toothed Club Moss, Wolf's Claw

Botanical Name:
Lycopodium clavatum

Common Uses:
Eczema, Psoriasis, Wound Care

Traditional Use:
The spores of the club moss have been used in traditional external skin washes for relief from the symptoms of eczema, psoriasis, and contact dermatitis.

Part Used:
Spores

Side Effects:
Club Moss is not recommended for use by women who are pregnant or nursing.

Club Moss is not recommended for use in children's treatments.

Club Moss is not recommended for use by people with asthma, pulmonary disease, seizures, or ulcers.

Club Moss may cause dizziness or nausea in some people.

The leaves and stems are toxic and should not be used in any treatment. The spores do not contain the toxins.

Additional uses and side effects may exist but further research is necessary to determine the exact properties and effects of use.

General:
Club moss is found worldwide and the spores of the club moss are harvested, dried and powdered for traditional inclusion in tea or added to traditional tinctures at a rate of 50 micrograms a day.

Coconut Oil
Coco Palm, Coconut Palm, Coconut Oil

Botanical Name:
Cocos nucifera

Common Uses:
Natural Skin Care

Traditional Use:
Coconut oil is a light oil that softens and heals skin making it suitable for all skin and hair types. It creates a natural foaming action when used in skin and hair care treatments.

Coconut oil helps to exfoliate the outer layer of dead skin cells and may reduce fine lines and wrinkles and smooth the skin.

Part Used:
Seed Meat, Oil

Side Effects:
Coconut is not recommended for use beyond dietary by women who are pregnant or nursing.

Coconut oil may raise cholesterol or weight.

Additional uses and side effects may exist but further research is necessary to determine the exact properties and effects of use.

General:
Coconut Oil is extracted from the nut of the coconut palm and is used in cooking, skin care, and traditional supplements.

Comfrey
Ass Ear, Black root, Blackwort, Comfrey, Gum Plant, Healing Herb, Knitback, Knitbone, Slippery Root, Wallwort

Botanical Name:
Symphytum officinale

Common Uses:
Eczema, Wound Healing

Traditional Use:

Comfrey tea is traditionally used as a skin wash for the treatment of eczema, skin sores, insect bites, hemorrhoids, and other skin disease and has been illustrated to speed wound healing but should only be applied to unbroken skin.

Part Used:
Leaf, Root

Side Effects:
Comfrey is not recommended for use by women who are pregnant or nursing.

Comfrey has shown toxicity effects and is for external use only.

Comfrey contains Pyrrolizidine Alkaloids with the root containing a higher amount than the leaves though either should be used with extreme caution in internal remedies.

Additional uses and side effects may exist but further research is necessary to determine the exact properties and effects of use.

General:
Comfrey is native to Europe, Asia, and the United States and the plants will self seed or can be started by root division or cuttings. The roots and leaves are harvested for fresh usage or dried and powdered for use in traditional treatments.

Cypress
Botanical Name:
Cupressus sempervirens

Common Uses:
Acne, Natural Skin Care

Traditional Use:
Cypress oil is used in to reduce excess oils in skin and hair care products and has been added to treatments for certain types of acne.

Cypress is known to tighten skin and refine the appearance of pores making it useful in facial care products.

Part Used:
Needles, Twigs

Side Effects:
Cypress is not recommended for use by women who are pregnant or nursing.

Additional uses and side effects may exist but further research is necessary to determine the exact properties and effects of use.

General:

Cypress is a well known essential oil native to Turkey but cultivated in other regions where the needles and twigs are harvested for their oil.

Damask Rose
Botanical Name:
Rosa damanscena

Common Uses:
Acne, Eczema, Natural Skin Care, Seborrhea

Traditional Use:
Damask Rose is included in natural skin care preparations to help clear the complexion, hydrate the skin and alleviate skin irritation like acne, eczema, and seborrhea.

Part Used:
Bud, Oil

Side Effects:
Additional uses and side effects may exist but further research is necessary to determine the exact properties and effects of use.

General:
Damask Rose is a deciduous member of the Rose family cultivated for rich rose scent. The shoots and buds are harvested and eaten as a raw or cooked vegetable while the petals have been used as a cooked jam component. The buds are harvested for use as a traditional supplement or the oils are extracted for use as an aromatherapy component

Dandelion
Blowball, Cankerwort, Clock Flower, Cochet, Dandelion, Dudhal, Endive, Fairy Clock, Fortune Teller, Irish Daisy, Lion's Tooth, Priest's Crown, Puff Ball, Swine Snout, Wild Endive

Botanical Name:
Taraxacum officinale

Common Uses:
Acne, Eczema, Psoriasis

Traditional Use:
Dandelion root helps the body to dispose of excess bacteria, toxins and hormones and has traditionally been used to help relieve skin conditions like acne, eczema, and psoriasis.

Part Used:
Leaf, Flower, Root

Side Effects:
Dandelion is not recommended for use by women who are pregnant or nursing.

Dandelion is not recommended for use by people with gall bladder disease without the guidance of a physician or qualified herbalist.

Dandelion is not recommended for use by people with stomach ulcers or gastritis.

Dandelion may cause stomach upset and diarrhea in some people.

Dandelion may cause an allergic reaction in some people.

General:
Dandelion is native to Asia, Europe, and North America where it is considered an invasive weed growing easily in a variety of sun, soil, and moisture conditions. It has been used by a variety of societies as a supplement treatment including the Native Americans. Dandelion leaf, flower, and root are used in salads, teas, and extracts and the flowers are sometimes used to make wine or in traditional teas up to 3 times daily.

Devils Bite
Devil's Bite, Gayfeather, Wildenow

Botanical Name:
Liatris scariosa

Common Uses:
Contact Dermatitis

Traditional Use:
Devils Bite has been used as a traditional topical poultice to alleviate the inflammation, itchiness, and pain associated with contact dermatitis, insect bites, and stings.

Part Used:
Rhizome – Root

Side Effects:
Devils Bite is not recommended for use by women who are pregnant or nursing.

Additional uses and side effects may exist but further research is necessary to determine the exact properties and effects of use.

General:
Devil's Bite is a perennial native to North America where it can be found growing wild in grasslands and open forest areas where the rhizomes are collected for use in a supplement alcohol extraction.

Dock – Bloody
Bloody Dock, Red Veined Dock

Botanical Name:
Rumex sanguineus

Common Uses:
Acne, Eczema, Psoriasis, Wound Care

Traditional Use:

Bloody Dock has been used as a traditional topical preparation to alleviate the symptoms of skin diseases like acne, eczema, and psoriasis.

Part Used:
Root

Side Effects:
Bloody Dock is not recommended for use by women who are pregnant or nursing.

Bloody Dock is not recommended for use by people with gout, rheumatism, arthritis, or kidney stones.

Additional uses and side effects may exist but further research is necessary to determine the exact properties and effects of use.

General:
Bloody Dock is a hardy perennial found growing in untended areas. The young leaves have been harvested for use as a cold or cooked vegetable and the leaves are harvested in the spring, dried and powdered for use in traditional supplements.

Dodder - Bigfruit
Botanical Name:
Cuscuta megalocarpa

Common Uses:
Contact Dermatitis

Traditional Use:
Big Fruit Dodder has been used as part of a traditional topical preparation to alleviate the discomfort associated with bites, stings, and contact dermatitis.

Part Used:
Threads

Side Effects:
Bigfruit Dodder is not recommended for use by women who are pregnant or nursing.

Bigfruit Dodder is not recommended for use by women who are trying to conceive as it has been used as a contraceptive in some cultures.

Additional uses and side effects may exist but further research is necessary to determine the exact properties and effects of use.

General:
Common Dodder is native to many tropical regions where it grows as a semi-parasitic plant on shrubs and herbs. The seed has been harvested for use as a flour product harvested, dried, and powdered for use as a traditional supplement.

Dog Rose
Botanical Name:
Rosa canina

130

Common Uses:
Natural Skin Care

Traditional Use:
Dog Rose hip infusions are used as an astringent wash for sensitive skin.

Part Used:
Hip

Side Effects:
Additional uses and side effects may exist but further research is necessary to determine the exact properties and effects of use.

General:
Dog Rose is a deciduous shrub cultivated in many regions of the world. The hips are harvested, eaten raw or cooked, used in jams & syrups, or made into a nutritive tea. The hips are also dried & powdered for use as a traditional topical or supplement preparation.

Edelweiss
Edelweiss, Lion's Paw, Queen's Flower
Botanical Name:
Leontopodium alpinum

Common Uses:
Natural Skin Care, Wound Care

Traditional Use:
Edelweiss contains anti-oxidants and sun screening properties making it a common ingredient in natural skin care products.

Edelweiss has traditionally been used in topical ointments to promote cell regeneration and speed wound healing.

Side Effects:
Additional uses and side effects may exist but further research is necessary to determine the exact properties and effects of use.

General:
Edelweiss can be found growing in higher altitudes and is cultivated as an ornamental for disinfectant and supplement uses.

Elderberry
Baccae, Black Elder, Elder, Elderberry, Ellanwood, Ellhorn, European Alder, Holunderbeeren, Sambucus, Sauco, Sureau

Botanical Name:
Sambucus nigra

Common Uses:
Acne, Natural Skin Care

Traditional Use:

Elderberry has been used as part of a traditional supplement to help detoxify the body and alleviate skin conditions like acne.

Elderberry is used as part of natural skin care products to detoxify and tone the skin while helping to fight aging.

Part Used:
Berry

Side Effects:
Elderberry is not recommended for use by women who are pregnant or nursing.

Unripe or uncooked elder berries are toxic and may cause nausea, vomiting, and diarrhea.

Additional uses and side effects may exist but further research is necessary to determine the exact properties and effects of use.

General:
Elder is native to Europe and North America but has been cultivated in other regions. The dried flowers and cooked berries of the elder are traditionally used in teas, extracts, and capsule form with a traditional infusion preparation being 2 teaspoon of dried flower to 1-cup boiling water 8 times daily.

Elder – Mexican
Botanical Name:
Sambucus mexicana

Common Uses:
Acne, Natural Hair & Skin Care

Traditional Use:
Mexican Elder flowers have been used as part of a traditional facial wash to alleviate acne outbreaks.

Part Used:
Flower, Root

Side Effects:
Mexican Elder is not recommended for use by women who are pregnant or nursing.

Mexican Elder may cause gastrointestinal upset.

Additional uses and side effects may exist but further research is necessary to determine the exact properties and effects of use.

General:
Mexican Elder is a deciduous shrub native to southern United States and Mexico where the flowers and fruit are harvested for use as a cooked or raw food product. The fruits and stems are used as dye products and the flower & root are harvested for use in traditional supplements.

Elecampane

Alant, Aster, Elecampane, Elfdock, Elfwort, Horse Elder, Horseheal, Indian Elecampane, Scabwort, Velvet Dock, Wild Sunflower, Yellow Starwort

Botanical Name:
Inula helenium

Common Uses:
Acne, Contact Dermatitis, Poison Ivy

Traditional Use:
Powdered Elecampane is traditionally added to a wash for the treatment of many eruptive skin diseases including acne, poison ivy, and boils.

Part Used:
Flower, Rhizome, Root

Side Effects:
Elecampane is not recommended for use by women who are pregnant or nursing.

Elecampane may cause allergies to people sensitive to plants in the sunflower family.

Elecampane may irritate the mucus membranes.

Elecampane may affect blood sugar.

Additional uses and side effects may exist but further research is necessary to determine the exact properties and effects of use.

General:
Elecampane is a perennial native to Europe and growing 4-6 feet in height that was naturalized to North America by the colonists and grows easily from root cuttings or seed. Elecampane prefers partial sunlight and moderate to highly moist soil. The root is harvested in the autumn, air dried, and ground or made in an alcohol extract for inclusion in traditional supplement preparations.

Elm - Indian

Indian Elm, Moose Elm, Orme Gras, Red Elm, Slippery Elm, Sweet Elm

Botanical Name:
Ulmus fulva

Common Uses:
Acne, Contact Dermatitis, Eczema, Wound Care

Traditional Use:
Indian Elm is traditionally included in topical ointments to draw impurities, reducing the appearance of acne and to treat eczema.

Indian Elm has a high mucilage content making it a traditional balm or poultice for burned, sun damaged, or irritated skin.

Indian Elm has been used as a traditional topical poultice to help speed healing in skin ulcers and wounds. It acts as a drawing ingredient to draw splinters, fragments, and infection away from the skin.

Part Used:
Flower, Inner Bark, Leaf

Side Effects:
Indian Elm is not recommended for use by women who are pregnant or nursing.

Indian Elm bark was once moistened and inserted into the vagina to cause cervical dilation and induce abortions.

Indian Elm may cause an allergic reaction.

Additional uses and side effects may exist but further research is necessary to determine the exact properties and effects of use.

General:
Indian Elm is native to North America and mature trees contain the highest level of active ingredients. The mature bark is harvested, dried, and ground fine for use in traditional supplement teas at a typical rate of rate of 2 tablespoons of powder to 1 cup of hot water or base up to 3 times daily. Chopped root or liquid extracts are more commonly used in poultice preparations.

Embauba

Embauba, Snakewood Tree, Trumpet Tree
Botanical Name:
Cecropia peltata

Common Uses:
Natural Skin Care

Traditional Use:
Embauba is used as a natural skin care ingredient and is traditionally believed to act as an anti-oxidant helping to reduce the effects of environmental aging and as an emollient to keep skin soft & supple.

Part Used:
Leaf, Resin

Side Effects:
Embauba is not recommended for use by women who are pregnant or nursing.

Embauba may have abortifacient effects.

Embauba is believed to affect the heart and is not recommended for use without the advice of a physician or qualified herbalist.

Embauba may affect blood sugar.

Additional uses and side effects may exist but further research is necessary to determine the exact properties and effects of use.

General:
Embauba is a small, fast growing tree native to tropical and sub-tropical regions and cultivated as an ornamental in frost-free zones. The wood is used as a lightweight craft product, the inner bark is used as a fiber product and the leaves are harvested for use as natural sandpaper. The young buds are harvested for use as a cooked vegetable and the leaf & resin are used in traditional supplements.

Ephedra - Torrey
Ephedra, Mexican Tea, Torrey Ephedra

Botanical Name:
Ephedra torreyana

Common Uses:
Eczema, Psoriasis

Traditional Use:
Torrey Ephedra has been used as a traditional topical lotion to alleviate itchiness and plaque formation in skin conditions like eczema and psoriasis.

Part Used:
Leaf, Stem

Side Effects:
The FDA banned the U.S. sale of dietary supplements containing ephedra. The FDA found that these supplements had a high risk of injury or illness and a risk of death. The ban does not apply to traditional Chinese herbal remedies or to products like herbal teas that are regulated as conventional foods.

Torrey Ephedra should only be used under the guidance of a physician or qualified herbalist.

Torrey Ephedra is not recommended for use by women who are pregnant or nursing.

Torrey Ephedra affects the brain and central nervous system in the same way as amphetamines but not as powerfully.

Torrey Ephedra is not recommended for use by people who have high blood pressure, hyperthyroidism, or glaucoma or who are taking MOAI inhibitors.

Torrey Ephedra works as a stimulant; it affects the heart and blood pressure. Due to the side effects, Ephedra has lost much of its appeal as a supplement.

Additional uses and side effects may exist but further research is necessary to determine the exact properties and effects of use.

General:

Torrey Ephedra is an evergreen shrub native to semi-desert and desert regions of the United States and Mexico. The stem and leaves of the ephedra plant are traditionally used in teas, extracts, tinctures and capsule form.

Epimedium
Barrenwort, Epimedium, Horny Goat Weed, Yin Yang Huo

Botanical Name:
Epimedium grandiflorum

Common Uses:
Anti-Aging

Traditional Use:
According to the Chinese Academy of Medical Science, epimedium slows down aging and promotes longevity.

Part Used:
Flower, Leaf, Seed

Side Effects:
Epimedium is not recommended for use by women who are pregnant or nursing.

Epimedium may lower blood pressure and may affect blood sugar.

Long-term use of Epimedium may cause dizziness, dry mouth, nosebleeds, spasms, thirst, and trouble breathing.

Overdoses of Epimedium can cause rapid heart rate, and high blood pressure. Standard Chinese Pharmaceutical dosages equal 6 mg of powder or 300 mg of dried leaf per 24-hour period.

Additional uses and side effects may exist but further research is necessary to determine the exact properties and effects of use.

General:
Epimedium is native to China, Japan, and Tibet but has become a popular landscape groundcover in other regions of the world. The flower, leaf, and seed have been harvested for thousands of years for use in traditional supplement preparations and have recently become popular in a variety of commercial pharmaceuticals and supplements.

Evening Primrose
Evening Primrose, Night Willow, Sundrop

Botanical Name:
Oenothera biennis

Common Uses:
Aging, Eczema, Natural Hair & Skin Care, Psoriasis, Seborrhea

Traditional Use:
Evening Primrose Oil has shown an ability to reduce premature aging and help heal damaged skin.

Evening Primrose oils and powder are used in traditional topical preparations to alleviate itching and redness of the skin including those associated with eczema, psoriasis, seborrhea and wounds.

Part Used:
Leaf, Seed Oil

Side Effects:
Evening Primrose is not recommended for use by women who are pregnant or nursing.

Evening Primrose is not recommended for use by people who have a bleeding disorder, seizures, schizophrenia or an immuno-sensitive disorder like Multiple Sclerosis or Lupus.

Evening Primrose can cause stomach upset, bloating, and headaches in some people.

Additional uses and side effects may exist but further research is necessary to determine the exact properties and effects of use.

General:
Evening primrose is Native to North America and naturalized to parts of Europe where the leaves and roots are harvested in the spring and eaten as a cold vegetable. The flowers and leaves are harvested, dried, and powdered for use in traditional supplements. The oil is extracted from the seeds harvested at the beginning of the flowering season. It grows easily from seed in a variety of soil, sun, and moisture conditions.

Fennel
Biri Sanuf, Bitter Fennel, Carosella, Fennel, Hinojo, Sweet Fennel, Wild Fennel, Xiao Hui Xiang

Botanical Name:
Foeniculum vulgare

Courage, Strength

Protection, Strength

Common Uses:
Acne, Natural Skin Care

Traditional Use:
Fennel has been used as a traditional supplement to increase urinary output and to help remove toxins from the body alleviating conditions like acne, gout, rheumatism and as a general detoxification agent.

Fennel oils have a natural cleansing and toning effect on the skin and are used in natural products to combat oil, fight wrinkles, and brighten the complexion.

Part Used:
Leaf, Oil, Root, Seed, Whole

Side Effects:
Fennel is not recommended for use by women who are pregnant or nursing.

Fennel is a uterine stimulant.

Fennel may cause photosensitivity, indigestion, pulmonary edema, and vomiting.

Fennel is not recommended for use by women who have an estrogen sensitive disorder like endometriosis, fibroids or certain types of cancer.

Additional uses and side effects may exist but further research is necessary to determine the exact properties and effects of use.

General:
Fennel is an annual plant native to the Mediterranean but is cultivated worldwide as it is easily grown from seed in rich soil with plenty of sun and moderate moisture. It grows to a height of 3-6 feet and has yellow flowers that bloom in the summer months. Fennel is harvested for use as a flavoring in beverages or dried and powdered for use in traditional supplements. The oils are extracted from the crushed seed for use in topical and aromatherapy treatments.

Fenugreek
Bird's Foot, Bockshornklee, Fenugreek, Greek Clover, Greek Hay

Botanical Name:
Trigonella foenum-graecum

Common Uses:
Eczema, Natural Hair & Skin Care, Skin Inflammation

Traditional Use:
Fenugreek is traditionally used in topical poultices designed for the relief of the symptoms of eczema, skin ulcers, and other skin inflammations.

Part Used:
Seed

Side Effects:
Fenugreek is not recommended for use by women who are pregnant or nursing.

Fenugreek is not recommended for use in children's treatments.

Fenugreek can cause gas, bloating, and diarrhea in some people.

Fenugreek can cause congestion, coughing, swelling and wheezing in some people.

Fenugreek may lower blood sugar.

Fenugreek may cause an allergic reaction or irritate the skin.

Fenugreek may interfere with the absorption of prescription medication.

Additional uses and side effects may exist but further research is necessary to determine the exact properties and effects of use.

General:
Use of fenugreek dates back to ancient Egypt and it is native to the Mediterranean. It has been cultivated in almost most regions of the world, where the ripe seeds are dried, ground, and eaten, used in a traditional supplement tea, or made into a paste for topical applications.

Field Scabious
Bluebuttons, Devil's Bit, Field Scabious, Gypsy's Rose

Botanical Name:
Knautia arvensis

Common Uses:
Eczema, Psoriasis, Wound Care

Traditional Use:
Field Scabious has traditionally been used as a tea tonic to promote faster healing and treat the symptoms of chronic or severe skin conditions like eczema, anal fissures, psoriasis, skin ulcers and wound care.

Part Used:
Flower, Leaf, Stem

Side Effects:
Field Scabious is not recommended for use by women who are pregnant or nursing.

Additional uses and side effects may exist but further research is necessary to determine the exact properties and effects of use.

General:
Field Scabious is found in nearly every region except the northernmost and southernmost parts of the world. It can be found growing in untended areas where the above ground parts are harvested, dried, and powdered for use in a traditional tea infusion.

Figwort
Carpenter's Square, Figwort, Heal All, Scorphula

Botanical Name:
Scrophularia nodosa

Common Uses:
Acne, Detoxification, Eczema, Psoriasis, Wound Care

Traditional Use:
Figwort tea is traditionally used a detoxifier to reduce acne, eczema, and psoriasis outbreaks.

Figwort is a traditional ingredient in ointments and poultices that reduce pain & inflammation and help speed healing in eczema, psoriasis, and wounds.

Part Used:
Flower, Leaf, Root, Stem

Side Effects:
Figwort is not recommended for use by women who are pregnant or nursing.

Figwort is not recommended for use by people with heart disease.

Figwort may affect blood sugar.

Additional uses and side effects may exist but further research is necessary to determine the exact properties and effects of use.

General:
Figwort is native to North America, Europe, and China where it is harvested before flowering for use as a tincture traditionally delivered at a rate of 15 drops up to 3 times a day.

Fireweed
Blood Vine, Blooming Sally, Flowering Willow, French Willow, Purple Rocket, Rosebay, Tame Withy, Wickup, Willow Herb

Botanical Name:
Chamerion angustifolium

Common Uses:
Acne, Wound Care

Traditional Uses:
Fireweed has been used in traditional topical washes, ointments, and poultices to help reduce inflammation and reduce the appearance of acne.

Fireweed is used as a topical preparation to help draw infection from wounds or foreign matter from wounds.

Parts Used:
Flower, Leaf, Stem

Side Effects:
Fireweed is not recommended for use by women who are pregnant or nursing.

Additional uses and side effects may exist but further research is necessary to determine the exact properties and effects of use.

General:

Fireweed is native to North America where the above ground parts are harvested early in the season for use as a candied product, tea substitute, or cold vegetable.

Fumitory
Beggary, Earth Smoke, Fumaria, Fumitory, Fumus, Hedge Fumitory, Vapor, Wax Dolls

Botanical Name:
Fumaria officinalis

Common Uses:
Acne, Dermatitis, Eczema, Natural Skin Care – Pigmentation, Psoriasis

Traditional Use:
Fumitory is traditionally used as a skin wash for clearing conditions like acne, eczema, and psoriasis.

Fumitory is used as a traditional supplement to detoxify the body and helps to clear skin conditions like acne, eczema, and psoriasis.

Fumitory is used as part of a traditional preparation to reduce hyper-pigmentation like age spots, freckles and dark scarring.

Part Used:
Flower, Leaf, Stem

Side Effects:
Fumitory is not recommended for use by women who are pregnant or nursing.

Overuse of Fumitory may cause diarrhea, trembling, convulsions and even death.

Additional uses and side effects may exist but further research is necessary to determine the exact properties and effects of use.

General:
Fumitory is native to Africa, Europe, and Siberia but has been naturalized to parts of North & South America where it is harvested for use as a grated, fresh supplement.

Galbanum
Botanical Name:
Ferula galbaniflua

Common Uses:
Natural Skin Care, Wound Care

Traditional Uses:
Galbanum oil has been used to help regenerate aged skin and provide hydration in natural skin care products.

Parts Used:
Bark, Root - Resin

Side Effects:
Additional uses and side effects may exist but further research is necessary to determine the exact properties and effects of use.

General:
Galbanum resin is harvested from the roots and trunk of the tree for use as a food flavoring, cosmetic fragrance, and traditional supplement

Galinsoga
Galinsoga, Gallant Soldier, Guasca, Mielcilla

Botanical Name:
Galinsoga parviflora

Common Uses:
Contact Dermatitis, Insect Bites - Stings, Wound Care

Traditional Use:
Galinsoga is used in traditional topical preparations to reduce the pain, inflammation, and itchiness associated with contact dermatitis and insect bites or stings.

Galinsoga juice is used as a topical wash to reduce bleeding and speed healing of minor wounds.

Part Used:
Flower, Leaf, Stem

Side Effects:
Additional uses and side effects may exist but further research is necessary to determine the exact properties and effects of use.

General:
Galinsoga is native to the Central America, South American and southwestern United States where it is considered an invasive weed by some. The leaves, stem, and shoots are harvested during flowering for use as a raw or cooked vegetable and seasoning product or juiced for use as a vegetable drink. The flowers, leaves, and stems are also harvested & juiced or used whole as part of traditional supplements.

Garlic Mustard
Botanical Name:
Alliaria petiolata

Common Uses:
Acne, Eczema, Wounds

Traditional Use:
Garlic Mustard has been used as a traditional detoxification to remove impurities and reduce the number and severity of acne and eczema attacks.

Garlic Mustard has been used as a traditional topical

poultice or ointment to clean and speed healing in skin ulcers, wounds, and sores.

Part Used:
Leaf, Seed

Side Effects:
Additional uses and side effects may exist but further research is necessary to determine the exact properties and effects of use.

General:
Garlic Mustard is native to Africa and Asia but has been naturalized to Europe and North America where it is considered an invasive species by some. The young leaves are harvested as a seasoning or raw vegetable. The seeds are harvested for use in traditional supplements.

Geranium
Botanical Name:
Pelargonium graveolens

Common Uses:
Acne, Anti-Aging, Contact Dermatitis, Eczema, Natural Skin & Hair Care, Wound Care

Traditional Use:
Geranium has analgesic, anti-inflammatory, antimicrobial, astringent, and styptic properties that make it a traditional treatment for minor abrasions, cuts, & burns and for natural skin care remedies to treat acne, eczema, and contact dermatitis.

Germanium oil is used in natural skin care products for its effect on mature skin and the radiant glow it leaves on all skin types.

Part Used:
Leaf, Oil

Side Effects:
Geranium is not recommended for use, even in topical preparations, by women who are pregnant or nursing.

Geranium oil may cause an allergic reaction or skin irritation in some people.

Additional uses and side effects may exist but further research is necessary to determine the exact properties and effects of use.

General:

Geranium is native to South Africa but has been cultivated as an annual landscape herb in many other countries and is easily propagated by cuttings or seed. The oils are extracted from the leaves and stems through steam distillation and used in traditional inhalant therapy, supplements, and perfumes.

Golden Seal
Eye Balm, Eye Root, Goldenroot, Goldenseal, Ground Raspberry, Indian Dye, Indian Plant, Indian Turmeric, Jaundice Root, Orange Root, Turmeric Root, Wild Curcuma, Yellow Indian Pain, Yellow Puccoon, Yellow Root

Botanical Name:
Hydrastis canadensis

Common Uses:
Acne, Eczema, Psoriasis, Wound Care

Traditional Use:
Goldenseal is traditionally used in topical antiseptic and antibacterial ointments for minor abrasions, cuts, and open wounds. The ointment will also be anti-inflammatory and has been used as a traditional topical preparation in the treatment of skin conditions like acne and eczema.

Golden seal is traditionally used to cleanse the body of toxins including excess uric acid and toxins related to conditions like acne, gout & rheumatism.

Part Used:
Leaf, Root, Underground Stem

Side Effects:
Goldenseal is not recommended for use by women who are pregnant or nursing.

Goldenseal is not recommended for use in children's treatments.

Goldenseal is not intended for long-term use.

Goldenseal contains alkaloids that are toxic in large doses.

Overdose of goldenseal can cause vomiting, diarrhea, or stomach upset in some people.

Goldenseal may lower blood sugar levels, raise blood pressure, or gastrointestinal upset.

Goldenseal may change the way your body reacts to other prescription drugs.

Additional uses and side effects may exist but further research is necessary to determine the exact properties and effects of use.

General:

Goldenseal is native to North America and can be found growing wild in part of the US or cultivated in many supplement gardens. The leaf and the underground stem and root of the Goldenseal plant are harvested, dried, and powdered for use in supplement teas or made into an extract.

Goose Grass
Goose Grass, Moor Grass, Prince's Feather, Silverweed, Trailing Tansy, Wild Agrimony

Botanical Name:
Potentilla anserina

Common Uses:
Contact Dermatitis, Seborrhea, Skin Inflammation

Traditional Uses:
Goose Grass is traditionally applied to the skin to help reduce inflammation and irritation and helps to dry out sores in contact dermatitis like poison ivy.

Goose Grass tea has been used as a traditional skin cleansing lotion helping to alleviate inflammation, redness, and seborrhea.

Goose Grass has traditionally been bruised and applied directly to skin ulcers and hemorrhoids to alleviate pain & inflammation, reduce seepage & bleeding, and speed healing.

Parts Used:
Flower, Leaf

Side Effects:
Goose Grass is not recommended for use by women who are pregnant or nursing.

Additional uses and side effects may exist but further research is necessary to determine the exact properties and effects of use.

General:
Goose Grass grows worldwide and can be found growing in nearly every soil, sun & moisture conditions where some consider it an invasive weed. The root is harvested and eaten as a raw or cooked vegetable or dried & powdered for use as a thickening & flour product while the leaves are harvested early in the season for use fresh or dried in traditional supplements.

Gotu Kola
Brahma Buti, Centellase, Divya, Gotu Kola, Indian Pennywort, White Rot

Botanical Name:
Centella asiatica

Common Uses:
Acne, Contact Dermatitis, Eczema, Natural Hair & Skin Care, Psoriasis, Scar Reduction, Wound Care

Traditional Use:
Gotu Kola is an astringent and anti-inflammatory making it a traditional ingredient in skin care washes for the treatment of acne, eczema, psoriasis, and contact dermatitis.

Gotu Kola has traditionally been used as a balm to help sooth burns, skin ulcers, and wounds while speeding healing.

Gotu Kola is traditionally used to speed wound healing, stimulate collagen production, and helps reduce scarring from acne and wounds.

Gotu Kola tea is used in natural skin care products to strengthen and rejuvenate the skin, hair, and nails by stimulating collagen synthesis.

Part Used:
Leaf, Stem

Side Effects:
Gotu Kola is not recommended for use by women who are pregnant or nursing.

Gotu Kola is not recommended for use by people with liver disease.

High doses of Gotu Kola may cause nausea, rash, and possibly liver damage.

Do not use Gotu Kola if you are taking prescription drugs to treat depression, high cholesterol, or high blood pressure.

Additional uses and side effects may exist but further research is necessary to determine the exact properties and effects of use.

General:
Gotu Kola is native to Asia, Africa, North America and South America where it can be found growing in moist areas. The whole plant is harvested, dried in full sun, and used in traditional supplement teas and as a liquid extract up to 3 times daily.

Grapefruit
Agume, Grapefruit, Shaddock

Botanical Name:
Citrus paradisi

Common Uses:
Acne, Natural Hair & Skin Care, Preservative

Traditional Use:
Grapefruit seed oil is traditionally used in natural hair & skin care products to reduce oil, tone the skin and in treatments for some types of acne.

Grapefruit oil acts as a natural preservative in

homemade cosmetics and supplements helping to extend their shelf life.

Part Used:
Fruit, Rind, Seed

Side Effects:
Grapefruit is not recommended for use beyond dietary in women who are pregnant or nursing.

Grapefruit may change the way that the body uses estrogen and is not recommended for use by menopausal women or by those who have an estrogen related condition like fibroids, endometriosis or certain types of cancer.

Grapefruit oil may cause photosensitivity.

Additional uses and side effects may exist but further research is necessary to determine the exact properties and effects of use.

Grape
Calzin, Draksha, Grape, Grape Seed, Grapeseed, Red Vine, Uva

Botanical Name:
Vitis vinifera

Branch, Leaf, Seed: Anti-Inflammatory, Anti-Viral, Astringent, Colorant, Diuretic, Emollient, Vasodilator

Common Uses:
Natural Hair & Skin Care

Traditional Use:
Grapeseed oil has emollient, regenerative and toning properties and is often used as a carrier oil in natural skin and hair care

Part Used:
Fruit, Leaf, Seed - Oil

Side Effects:
Grape is not recommended for use beyond dietary by women who are pregnant or nursing.

Grape seed may cause dizziness, dry scalp, high blood pressure, hives, indigestion, nausea, sore throat, stomach upset, and vomiting.

Additional uses and side effects may exist but further research is necessary to determine the exact properties and effects of use.

General:
The leaves, branches, and fruits of the grape have been used as a supplement since the time of the Ancient Greeks and the grapes used to produce grape seed extract are typically obtained from wine manufacturers.

The roots of another species of grape the wild grape, Vitis riparia roots yield a purple colorant.

Green Osier
Agoda Dogwood, Green Osier

Botanical Name:
Cornus alternifolia

Common Uses:
Acne, Contact Dermatitis, Eczema, Wound Care

Traditional Use:
Green Osier barks has traditionally been used as a powder or wash to reduce inflammation and help speed the healing of acne, blisters, eczema, and wounds.

Part Used:
Bark

Side Effects:
Additional uses and side effects may exist but further research is necessary to determine the exact properties and effects of use.

General:
Green Osier is native to North America where it has been used as a dye product and traditional supplement for thousands of years.

Grindelia
Grindelia, Gum plant, Tarweed

Botanical Name:
Grindelia robusta

Common Uses:
Contact Dermatitis

Traditional Use:
Grindelia has an anti-inflammatory and antibacterial action that makes it a traditional treatment for skin inflammations like contact dermatitis, insect bites, and poison ivy rashes.

Part Used:
Flower, Leaf, Stem

Side Effects:
Grindelia is not recommended for use by women who are pregnant or nursing.

Overuse of Grindelia may cause gastrointestinal upset.

Grindelia may have an effect on the heart and should be used under the guidance of a physician or qualified herbalist.

Additional uses and side effects may exist but further research is necessary to determine the exact properties and effects of use.

General:
Grindelia is native to Central and North America and can be grown by cuttings or seed. It does well in poor quality, alkaline soils where other plants may have difficulty thriving. The leaf and flowers are harvested before the buds open, dried in full sunlight, powdered, and incorporated into traditional supplement infusions up to 3 times daily.

Guava
Amrood, Fan Shi Liu, Goyabe, Guava

Botanical Name:
Psidium guajava

Common Uses:
Contact Dermatitis, Wound Care

Traditional Uses:
Guava bark has traditionally been added to bath water to alleviate the irritation and inflammation of contact dermatitis and other itchy skin conditions.

Parts Used:
Bark, Fruit, Leaf

Side Effects:
Guava is not recommended for use beyond dietary by women who are pregnant or nursing.

Overuse of Guava may cause diarrhea.

Additional uses and side effects may exist but further research is necessary to determine the exact properties and effects of use.

General:
Guava is a tropical fruit native to Brazil, Columbia, Mexico and Venezuela where the fruit is eaten, made into beverages and harvested along with the leaves for use in traditional supplements.

Guggul
Guggul, Koushika, Mukul Myrrh Tree

Botanical Name:
Commiphora wightii

Common Uses:
Acne

Traditional Uses:
Guggul has been used as a traditional supplement tea to help alleviate some types of acne and eczema outbreaks. Studies show that it may work as well as prescription antibiotics to reduce the number and severity of acne outbreaks.

Parts Used:
Resin

Side Effects:
Guggul is not recommended for use by women who are pregnant or nursing.

Guggul is not recommended for use by people who have a hormone sensitive condition like endometriosis, fibroids, or cancer.

Guggul is not recommended for use by people who have a thyroid condition.

Guggul may cause diarrhea, headaches, nausea, vomiting, or skin rashes in some people.

Additional uses and side effects may exist but further research is necessary to determine the exact properties and effects of use.

General:
Guggal is made from the gum resin of the Indian Mukul Tree. Guggal is cultivated for the gummy resin. It is harvested for use as a perfumery and incense similar to myrrh. The resin of Guggal has been used in traditional supplements since ancient times.

Gum Dragon
Adragante, Goat's Thorn, Green Dragon, Gum Dragon, Gummi Tragacanthae, Gum Tragacanth, Hog Gum, Tragacanto

Botanical Name:
Astragalus gummifera , Syrian Tragacanth

Common Uses:
Natural Care Products

Traditional Uses:
Dragon gum is used as a binding and thickening agent in toothpaste, hand lotion, creams, ointments, and jelly.

Parts Used:
Gum Resin

Side Effects:
Dragon Gum is not recommended for use beyond dietary by women who are pregnant or nursing.

Dragon Gum may cause an allergic reaction in some people.

Additional uses and side effects may exist but further research is necessary to determine the exact properties and effects of use.

General:
Gum Dragon is a plant whose resin is used as a cold-water stabilizing and thickening agent in foods, pharmaceuticals, and personal care products. The resin is also used in supplement preparations.

Gumbo Limbo
Botanical Name:

140

Bursera simaruba

Common Uses:
Contact Dermatitis

Traditional Use:
Gumbo Limbo resin been used as part of a traditional topical preparation to reduce inflammation and itchiness associated with contact dermatitis like poison ivy.

Part Used:
Leaf

Side Effects:
Additional uses and side effects may exist but further research is necessary to determine the exact properties and effects of use.

General:
Gumbo Limbo is native to Central America, southern North America, and South America. It is easily grown from cuttings and cultivated as wind resistant hedge lines. The wood is used for craftwork and the resin is used as a glue or varnish product.

Hairy Agrimony
Botanical Name:
Agrimonia pilosa

Common Uses:
Eczema, Psoriasis

Traditional Use:
Hairy Agrimony has been used as part of a traditional topical preparation and supplement treatment to reduce the number and severity of skin conditions like eczema and psoriasis.

Side Effects:
Hairy Agrimony is not recommended for use by women who are pregnant or nursing.

Hairy Agrimony may lower blood sugar.

Additional uses and side effects may exist but further research is necessary to determine the exact properties and effects of use.

General:
Hairy Agrimony is a perennial cultivated in many regions of the world as an ornamental. The leaves are harvested and eaten as a cooked vegetable while the seeds are harvested, dried and powdered for use as flour. The leaves are harvested at the beginning of the flowering season, dried, and powdered for use in traditional supplements.

Hairy Sage
Hairy Sage, Herba Schizonepatae, Japanese Catnip, Japanese Mint, Jing Jie, Tenuifolia

Botanical Name:
Schizonepeta multifida

Common Uses:
Contact Dermatitis, Eczema, Psoriasis

Traditional Uses:
Hairy Sage has traditionally been used to reduce the symptoms of contact dermatitis, eczema, and psoriasis.

Parts Used:
Leaf, Stem

Side Effects:
Hairy Sage is not recommended for use by women who are pregnant or nursing.

Hairy Sage is not recommended for use by people who have liver disease.

Additional uses and side effects may exist but further research is necessary to determine the exact properties and effects of use.

Harts Tongue
Buttonhole, God's Hair, Hind's Tongue, Horse Tongue

Botanical Name:
Asplenium scolopendrium

Common Uses:
Acne, Natural Hair & Skin Care

Traditional Uses:
Harts tongue fronds have been used in natural hair & skin care washes to reduce oils and is traditionally believed to reduce acne.

Parts Used:
Leaf, Stem

Side Effects:
Harts tongue is not recommended for use by women who are pregnant or nursing.

Harts tongue is not recommended for long-term use.

Additional uses and side effects may exist but further research is necessary to determine the exact properties and effects of use.

General:
Harts tongue is an evergreen groundcover and harvested for use in natural hair & skin care products or traditional supplements.

Hawthorn
Aubepine, Haw, Hawthorne, Maybush, Maythorn, Whitehorn

Botanical Name:
Crataegus laevigata

Common Uses:
Acne, Eczema, Psoriasis

Traditional Uses:
Hawthorn berries have been used as a traditional treatment to reduce impurities and alleviate skin conditions like acne, eczema, and psoriasis.

Parts Used:
Berry, Flower, Leaf

Side Effects:
Hawthorn is not recommended for use by women who are pregnant or nursing.

Hawthorn is not recommended for use by people on medication for heart disease, blood pressure, or who have a condition related to heart or blood pressure. Hawthorn may change the way the body reacts to medications including digitalis.

Hawthorn can cause agitation, dizziness, fatigue, headache, insomnia, nausea, nosebleeds, and other problems in some people.

Additional uses and side effects may exist but further research is necessary to determine the exact properties and effects of use.

General:
Hawthorn is native to temperate northern regions where it has been used for hundreds of years as a food and traditional supplement. The berries, flowers, and leaves all contain active cardiac compounds but the most effect is found in the leaves harvested during the flowering season. Hawthorn is harvested, dried & powdered or available in commercial supplements.

Hazel
Aveleira, Cobnut, Hazel, Hazel Nut, Noisettes

Botanical Name:
Corylus avellana

Common Uses:
Carrier Oil, Natural Skin Care

Traditional Uses:
Hazelnut Oil is traditionally used in oily or combination natural hair & skin care products for its ability to tone and tighten the skin while promoting cell regeneration and infusing moisture.

Hazelnut has been used as a traditional dietetic additive to help lower cholesterol.

Hazelnut bark, roots, and nuts yield colorants in shades of brown to tan.

Hazelnut oil is traditionally used to treat intestinal parasites like threadworm.

Parts Used:
Bark, Leaf, Nut – Oil

Side Effects:
Hazelnut is not recommended for use beyond dietary by women who are pregnant or nursing.

Hazelnut may cause an allergic reaction in some people.

Additional uses and side effects may exist but further research is necessary to determine the exact properties and effects of use.

General:
Hazelnuts are the fruit of the hazel tree and are harvested as a food. Nuts are eaten whole, dried & powdered as a flour product, or included as a flavoring in drinks and foods. The nuts are also harvested for oil extraction and used as traditional supplements.

Hearts Ease
Field Pansy, Heartsease, Heart's Ease, Johnny Jump In, Ladies Delight, Pansy, Pennsee, Viola, Wild Pansy

Botanical Name:
Viola tricolor

Common Uses:
Acne, Eczema, Psoriasis

Traditional Use:
Hearts Ease is most traditionally used as an external ointment to help heal chronic skin conditions including acne, cradle cap, eczema, impetigo, and psoriasis.

Part Used:
Flower, Leaf, Stem

Side Effects:
Hearts Ease is not recommended for use by women who are pregnant or nursing.

Additional uses and side effects may exist but further research is necessary to determine the exact properties and effects of use.

General:
Hearts Ease is a member of the viola family native to Asia and Europe and cultivated in other regions where it is harvested during the flowering season, dried, and powdered for use in ointments, shampoos and traditional supplement teas up to 3 times daily.

Heartseed Walnut
Heartseed Walnut, Japanese Walnut

Botanical Name:
Juglans ailanthifolia cordiformis

Common Uses:

Acne, Natural Skin Care, Wound Care

Traditional Use:
The oils of the heartseed walnut are used in natural skin care products giving a light astringent and toning effect traditionally used to combat acne while smoothing the overall texture of the skin.

The oils of the heartseed walnut are used as a traditional topical preparation to speed healing in skin ulcers and minor wounds.

Part Used:
Nut - Oil

Side Effects:
Additional uses and side effects may exist but further research is necessary to determine the exact properties and effects of use.

General:
Heart Seed Walnut is a deciduous tree native to Asia where the seeds are harvested for use as a raw or cooked food product or the oils extracted for use in cooking or cosmetics.

Heather
Culluna, Heather, Ling

Botanical Name:
Calluna vulgaris

Common Uses:
Acne

Traditional Use:
Heather has traditionally been used to detoxify the body and lessen the severity and number of acne outbreaks.

Part Used:
Flower, Leaf

Side Effects:
Heather is not recommended for use by women who are pregnant or nursing.

Additional uses and side effects may exist but further research is necessary to determine the exact properties and effects of use.

General:
Heather is an evergreen shrub like plant growing 12-18 inches in height but able to be cultivated into a hedge. Heather blooms in mid-summer with a variety of pink toned flowers. It has been naturalized to the east coast of North America where it harvested while in bloom, dried and used as a traditional supplement tea up to 3 times daily.

Hemp Agrimony
Botanical Name:

Eupatorium cannabinum

Common Uses:
Acne

Traditional Use:
Hemp Agrimony has traditionally been used to detoxify the body and minimize the episodes of conditions like acne, gout, and rheumatism.

Part Used:
Flower, Leaf

Side Effects:
Hemp Agrimony is not recommended for use by women who are pregnant or nursing.

Hemp Agrimony contains compounds that make it unsuitable for use without the guidance of a physician or qualified herbalist.

Overuse of Hemp Agrimony may cause diarrhea, vomiting, or liver damage.

Additional uses and side effects may exist but further research is necessary to determine the exact properties and effects of use.

General:
Hemp Agrimony is native to Asia but cultivated as an ornamental plant in other regions where the flower & leaf are harvested, dried, and powdered for use in traditional supplements.

Henna
Alcanna, Egyptian Privet, Henna, Mehndi, Mendee, Mignonette Tree, Reseda, Smooth Lawsonia

Botanical Name:
Lawsonia inermis

Common Uses:
Acne, Eczema, Natural Hair & Skin Care,

Traditional Use:
Henna has illustrated an ability to ease the discomfort and appearance of skin conditions including acne, eczema, and psoriasis.

Part Used:
Bark, Fruit, Leaf

Side Effects:
Henna is not recommended for use by women who are pregnant or nursing.

Henna has been used as a uterine stimulant and may have abortifacient properties.

Henna is not recommended for use in children's treatments.

Henna is not recommended for internal treatments without the advice of a physician or qualified herbalist.

Henna may cause an allergic reaction or skin irritation.

Additional uses and side effects may exist but further research is necessary to determine the exact properties and effects of use.

General:
Henna is native to the Middle East where it is harvested, dried, and powdered for use in external applications or as a traditional supplement tea up to 3 times daily.

Honey Locust
Botanical Name:
Gleditsia sinensis

Common Uses:
Acne, Eczema, Psoriasis, Wound Care

Traditional Use:
Honey Locust thorns & thorns have traditionally been used as an ointment or wash to help clean & speed healing in acne, eczema, psoriasis and eruptive skin diseases.

Honey Locust juice & thorns have been used as a traditional skin wash or ointment to clean and speed healing of skin ulcers, sores, and wounds.

Part Used:
Leaf, Seed, Thorn

Side Effects:
Honey Locust may contain toxic compounds and is not recommended for use without the advice of a physician or qualified herbalist.

Honey Locust is not recommended for use by women who are pregnant or nursing.

Additional uses and side effects may exist but further research is necessary to determine the exact properties and effects of use.

General:
Honey Locust is a deciduous tree native to Asia, Europe and North America where the seedpod has been harvested for use as a soap product, the seeds have been used as a sugar substitute, and the wood is used for construction. The leaf, seed, and thorn are harvested for use in traditional supplements.

Honeysuckle – Japanese
Botanical Name:
Lonicera japonica

Common Uses:
Acne

Traditional Use:

Japanese Honeysuckle flowers & leaves have been used as a traditional topical preparation to alleviate certain types of acne outbreaks.

Part Used:
Bark, Flower, Leaf

Side Effects:
Japanese Honeysuckle is not recommended for use by women who are pregnant or nursing.

Additional uses and side effects may exist but further research is necessary to determine the exact properties and effects of use.

General:
Japanese Honeysuckle is native to Asia and is commonly cultivated in many regions of the world as a fragrant and ornamental. Japanese Honeysuckle has been used in Chinese supplements for thousands of years. The leaves are harvested and eaten as a cooked vegetable while the flowers are used as a sweet syrup.

Horse Chestnut - Indian
Botanical Name:
Aesculus indica

Common Uses:
Acne, Eczema, Psoriasis

Traditional Use:
Indian Horse Chestnut oil has traditionally been used as a topical wash or ointment ingredient to alleviate acne, eczema, and psoriasis.

Part Used:
Seed - Oil

Side Effects:
Indian Horse Chestnut is not recommended for use by women who are pregnant or nursing.

Indian Horse Chestnuts are known to have narcotic properties and should not be used without the advice of a physician or qualified herbalist.

Additional uses and side effects may exist but further research is necessary to determine the exact properties and effects of use.

Houseleek
Ayegreen, Bullock's Eye, Hens and Chicks, Jupiter's Beard, Thunder Plant

Botanical Name:
Sempervivum tectorum

Common Uses:
Acne, Eczema, Psoriasis

Traditional Uses:

Houseleek has been used as a traditional topical or supplement preparation to alleviate itchy or eruptive skin conditions like acne, eczema, and psoriasis.

Houseleek is traditionally included as part of a topical ointment to cleanse and speed healing in burns, sores, skin ulcers, and wounds.

Houseleek juice has been used as a traditional topical preparation to remove warts & corns.

Parts Used:
Whole - Juice

Side Effects:
Houseleek is not recommended in women who are pregnant or nursing.

General:
Houseleeks are a form of evergreen succulent found in higher altitudes worldwide where they are cultivated in sunny rock gardens and for use as a traditional supplement. The plant is harvested and juiced for use in topical preparations and the leaves are used as part of a traditional supplement.

Hyacinth
Bai Qu, Hyacinth - Orchid

Botanical Name:
Bletia hyacinthina

Common Uses:
Acne, Eczema, Psoriasis, Skin Damage, Wounds

Traditional Use:
Hyacinth bulb is traditionally powdered for use in topical preparations to attract moisture, reduce itching & inflammation, and speed healing in conditions like acne, burns, eczema, psoriasis, skin damage, and wounds.

Part Used:
Bulb - Root

Side Effects:
Hyacinth is not recommended for use by women who are pregnant or nursing.

Additional uses and side effects may exist but further research is necessary to determine the exact properties and effects of use.

General:
Hyacinth is native to Japan but is also a common ornamental cultivated worldwide for its spring flowers. The bulb is used to add sheen to ink, polishes, and other products and as a traditional supplement.

Immortelle

Shrubby Everlasting, Eternal Flower, Goldilocks, Immortelle, Sandy Everlasting, Strawflower, Yellow Chaste Weed

Botanical Name:
Helichrysum angustifolium

Common Uses:
Anti-Aging, Natural Skin Care, Scar Reduction

Traditional Use:
Immortelle is believed to have regenerative properties that stimulate new skin cell production making it a common ingredient in skin care treatments especially for aged skin.

Immortelle is a traditional component in natural skin care treatments to reduce the appearance of cellulite and fade the appearance of hyperactive pigmentation, scarring, and stretch marks.

Part Used:
Flower

Side Effects:
Immortelle is not recommended for use by women who are pregnant or nursing.

Immortelle is not recommended for use in children's treatments.

Immortelle is not recommended for use by people who have a blocked bile duct or gallstones.

Immortelle may cause an allergic reaction in some people.

Additional uses and side effects may exist but further research is necessary to determine the exact properties and effects of use.

General:
Immortelle is native to Europe and the United States and is harvested as the buds begin to bloom. They are dried, powdered and used in traditional supplement teas up to 3 times daily. Immortelle oil is steam distilled within 24 hours of harvesting the flower for use in topical and aromatherapy preparations.

Impatiens
Balsam Weed, Impatiens, Jewel Weed, Jewelweed, Silverweed, Slipper Weed, Touch Me not, Wild Balsam, Wild Celandine

Botanical Name:
Impatiens capensis, Impatiens biflora

Common Uses:
Skin Care – Contact Dermatitis

Traditional Use:

Impatiens juice is a traditional remedy for the topical treatment of a variety of skin ailments. The leaves are crushed and rubbed on irritated skin resulting from poison ivy rashes, insect bites, and other eruptions from contact dermatitis.

Part Used:
Juice

Side Effects:
Impatiens is not recommended for use by women who are pregnant or nursing.

Impatiens is for external use only.

Additional uses and side effects may exist but further research is necessary to determine the exact properties and effects of use.

General:
Impatiens is native to North America and can be cultivated in partly shaded areas with high moisture where they are harvested and the juice extracted for use in external preparations.

Indian Coral
Flame Tree, Indian Coral, Kaffirboom

Botanical Name:
Erythrina variegata

Common Uses:
Acne, Eczema, Psoriasis, Wound Care

Traditional Use:
Indian Coral is used as a traditional topical preparation to reduce inflammation and speed healing of acne, eczema, psoriasis, wounds, and other inflammatory skin conditions.

Part Used:
Bark, Leaf

Side Effects:
Indian Coral is not recommended for use by women who are pregnant or nursing.

Additional uses and side effects may exist but further research is necessary to determine the exact properties and effects of use.

General:
Indian Coral is a flowering tree cultivated in tropical and subtropical regions for its showy flowers. The leaves and bark have been harvested for use in traditional topical and supplement preparations.

Indian Mallow
Abutilon, Dong Kui Zi, Indian Mallow

Botanical Name:
Abutilon indicum

Common Uses:
Acne, Wound Care

Traditional Use:
Indian Mallow has been used as a traditional topical poultice to reduce the pain & inflammation while speeding healing in acne, skin ulcers, and wounds.

Part Used:
Whole Plant – Bark, Flower, Leaf, Root, Stem

Side Effects:
This is not recommended for use by women who are pregnant or nursing.

Additional uses and side effects may exist but further research is necessary to determine the exact properties and effects of use.

General:
Indian Mallow is a shrub native to tropical and sub-tropical regions where it is cultivated as an ornamental and the whole plant is harvested, dried, and powdered for use as a traditional supplement infusion.

Indian Nettle
Cat's Nettle, Indian Nettle

Botanical Name:
Acalypha indica

Common Uses:
Contact Dermatitis, Eczema, Psoriasis

Traditional Use:
Indian nettle has been used as a traditional topical preparation to treat skin inflammation and irritation from contact dermatitis and to reduce the symptoms of eczema and psoriasis.

Part Used:
Whole

Side Effects:
Indian Nettle is not recommended for use by women who are pregnant or nursing.

Indian Nettle may cause an allergic reaction or skin irritation.

Indian Nettle contains small amounts of toxins and overuse may cause gastrointestinal upset, liver damage, or kidney damage.

General:
Indian Nettle is an annual herb native to the Middle East but cultivated in other areas. The leaf, roots, and stems are harvested during flowering, dried, and powdered for use in traditional supplements.

Indigo – Wild

American Indigo, Baptista, False Indigo, Horsefly Weed, Indigo Broom, Rattlebush, Wild Indigo, Yellow Indigo

Botanical Name:
Baptisia tinctoria

Common Uses:
Acne, Wound Care

Traditional Use:
Wild Indigo has traditionally been used as part of a topical ointment, wash, or poultice to treat infections like staphylococcus, reduce acne outbreaks, and speed healing in skin ulcers and wounds.

Part Used:
Root

Side Effects:
Wild Indigo is not recommended for use by women who are pregnant or nursing.

Wild Indigo is not recommended for use in children's treatments.

Wild Indigo is not recommended for people with gastrointestinal disorders.

Overuse of Wild Indigo may cause diarrhea, difficulty breathing, increased heart rate, nausea, vomiting or even death.

Additional uses and side effects may exist but further research is necessary to determine the exact properties and effects of use.

General:
Wild Indigo is native to North America where it can be found growing wild along the Eastern half of the country. It is harvested, dried and powdered for use in traditional supplement infusions up to 3 times daily or in ointment preparations at a rate of 1:1 in 60% alcohol.

Iris – Yellow
Iris, Yellow Flag, Yellow Iris

Botanical Name:
Iris pseudacorus

Common Uses:
Acne, Wound Care

Traditional Use:
Yellow Flag is traditionally used to reduce inflammation, pain, and speed healing in severe acne, skin ulcers, and wounds.

Part Used:
Root

Side Effects:

Yellow Iris is not recommended for use by women who are pregnant or nursing.

Yellow Iris may cause an allergic reaction or skin irritation.

Overuse of Yellow Iris may cause severe diarrhea and vomiting.

Additional uses and side effects may exist but further research is necessary to determine the exact properties and effects of use.

General:
Yellow Iris is a scented perennial cultivated as an ornamental in many regions of the world. The seed is harvested for use as a coffee substitute and the flowers & roots are used as a dye product. The root is used to make ink and in traditional supplements.

Irish Moss
Botanical Name:
Chondrus crispus

Common Uses:
Acne, Natural Hair & Skin Care Products, Skin Inflammation

Traditional Use:
Irish Moss has traditionally been used as a topical ointment or wash component to alleviate acne and skin inflammation.

Part Used:
Whole

Side Effects:
Irish Moss is not recommended for use by women who are pregnant or nursing.

Additional uses and side effects may exist but further research is necessary to determine the exact properties and effects of use.

General:
Irish Moss is a red algae that is collected from the coast of Ireland, washed, bleached in the sun, and powdered for use as a thickening agent, stabilizer, and as a traditional supplement infusion.

Ivy - English
English Ivy, Gum Ivy, Lierre Grimpant, True Ivy, Woodbind

Botanical Name:
Hedera helix

Common Uses:
Acne, Wound Care

Traditional Use:

English Ivy has been used in topical ointments and washes to help reduce the appearance of acne outbreaks.

Part Used:
Berry, Leaf

Side Effects:
English Ivy is not recommended for use by women who are pregnant or nursing.

English Ivy may cause an allergic reaction or gastrointestinal upset in some people.

Additional uses and side effects may exist but further research is necessary to determine the exact properties and effects of use.

General:
English ivy is native to Asia and Europe but has been naturalized to many areas of the world where it is harvested, dried, and powdered for use in external applications or traditional tea supplement up to 3 times daily.

Jambul
Badijamun, Black Plum, Duhat, Jambol, Jambul, Jambolan, Jambulan, Jamum, Java Plum, Phadena, Rose Apple

Botanical Name:
Eugenia jambolana

Common Uses:
Contact Dermatitis, Eczema, Psoriasis

Traditional Use:
Jambul has been approved for use in European Pharmaceuticals to treat eczema, psoriasis, and contact dermatitis.

Part Used:
Bark, Leaf, Seed

Side Effects:
Jambul is not recommended for use by women who are pregnant or nursing.

Jambul has an effect on blood sugar, monitor sugar levels carefully and do not use without consulting a physician or qualified herbalist.

Additional uses and side effects may exist but further research is necessary to determine the exact properties and effects of use.

General:
Jambul is native to India and Pakistan but has naturalized throughout much of China and Australia where the fruit is harvested for use as a cooked or raw food product. The fruit, seeds, and bark are also harvested and dried for use in traditional supplements

with a daily dosage of 30 seeds or as a decoction of 1 to 2 teaspoonfuls to 1 cup of water up to 3 times daily.

Jasmine
Jasmine, Jessamine

Botanical Name:
Jasminum officinale

Common Uses:
Natural Skin & Hair Care

Traditional Use:
Jasmine Oil is included in natural hair & skin care products to help tone dry or greasy skin and promote elasticity.

Part Used:
Flower, Oil – pick before dawn when oils are strongest

Side Effects:
Jasmine is not recommended for use by women who are pregnant or nursing.

Additional uses and side effects may exist but further research is necessary to determine the exact properties and effects of use.

General:
Jasmine is cultivated in many regions of the world as an ornamental plant but is also harvested for use as a traditional tea or oil supplement. Jasmine flower are traditionally harvested at dawn when the oils are strongest.

Jojoba
Deernut, Goatnut, Jojoba, Pignut

Botanical Name:
Simmondsia chinensis

Common Uses:
Acne, Carrier Oil, Natural Hair, Skin & Face Care, Preservative, Psoriasis

Traditional Use:
Jojoba helps to unclog the pores and dissolve excess sebum and is traditionally used in topical preparations to alleviate some types of acne.

Jojoba is a rich, moisturizing oil that resembles the sebum in human skin and is easily absorbed by the skin and does not cause irritation for most skin types making it a preferred oil for use in natural hair & skin care products.

Jojoba has been used as a natural preservative in supplements, food products, and cosmetics.

Part Used:
Leaf, Seed, Oil, Wax

Side Effects:
Jojoba Oil is for external use only and should not be ingested.

Jojoba may cause an allergic skin reaction in some people.

Additional uses and side effects may exist but further research is necessary to determine the exact properties and effects of use.

General:
Jojoba is native to the Deserts of North America and Latin America. The oil and wax produced by the Jojoba seed are used in natural care products and supplements.

Jurema
Botanical Name:
Mimosa hostilis

Common Uses:
Acne, Burns, Natural Skin Care, Wounds

Traditional Use:
Jurema is used in commercial and traditional skin care products to rejuvenate the skin, reduce acne, and combat aging.

Jurema is traditionally used in topical preparations to reduce pain, speed healing, and rejuvenate skin in injuries like burns, sores, ulcers, and wounds.

Part Used:
Leaf

Side Effects:
is not recommended for use by women who are pregnant or nursing.

Additional uses and side effects may exist but further research is necessary to determine the exact properties and effects of use.

General:
Jurema is an evergreen shrub native to Central America and South America where it has been harvested as a traditional supplement for thousands of years.

Juniper
Guinevere, Ginepro, Juniper, Juniper Berries, Zimbro

Botanical Name:
Juniperus communis

Common Uses:
Acne, Eczema, Psoriasis, Wound Care

Traditional Use:
Juniper oil has astringent and antiseptic properties that make it a traditional toning oil for acne treatments

while its stimulating properties have shown benefits in treating eczema and psoriasis.

Part Used:
Berry, Needles, Oil

Side Effects:
Juniper is not recommended for use by women who are pregnant or nursing.

Juniper is not recommended for use by people who have diabetes, intestinal disorders, high blood pressure or kidney disease.

Overuse may cause urine to smell like violets.

Overdose can cause kidney irritation, blood in the urine, and potential liver damage.

Juniper Oil is for external use only.

Additional uses and side effects may exist but further research is necessary to determine the exact properties and effects of use.

General:
Juniper is native to Africa, Asia, Europe and North America. Juniper berries are harvested for use as a diet or tea supplement while the oils are extracted from the needles. Do not bruise or crush the berries until you are ready to use them.

Kokum
Botanical Name:
Garcinia indica

Common Uses:
Contact Dermatitis, Eczema, Skin Irritation

Traditional Use:
Kokum leaves & bark have been used as a traditional infusion or topical preparation to alleviate skin irritation, eczema, and contact dermatitis.

Part Used:
Bark, Fruit, Leaf

Side Effects:
Kokum is not recommended for use by women who are pregnant or nursing.

Additional uses and side effects may exist but further research is necessary to determine the exact properties and effects of use.

General:
Kokum is a fruit bearing tree native to Africa, Asia, and India where it is cultivated for a variety of uses. The fruit is harvested as a food or drink product, the oils are harvested for use in foods, medicines, and cosmetics, and the bark, leaf, and fruit are used as commercial

pharmaceuticals, traditional supplements and dietary supplements.

Kombu
Kombu, Konbu

Botanical Name:
Laminaria japonica

Common Uses:
Natural Hair & Skin Care

Traditional Use:
Kombu has been used as a natural hair & skin care product to provide essential nutrition, remove toxins and give a silky smooth feel to the hair, lips, nails, and skin.

Part Used:
Whole

Side Effects:
Kombu is not recommended for use by women who are pregnant or nursing.

Kombu is not recommended for use by people with a thyroid disorder and may cause thyroid changes in others.

Kombu is not recommended for use by people who have a kidney disorder.

Additional uses and side effects may exist but further research is necessary to determine the exact properties and effects of use.

General:
Kombu is a seaweed cultivated in Asia for use as a nutritious food or harvested, dried, and powdered for use in traditional supplements.

Kukui Nut
Candlenut, Indian Walnut, Kukui Nut, Varnish Tree

Botanical Name:
Aleurites moluccanus

Common Uses:
Acne, Eczema, Mouth Natural Hair & Skin Care, Psoriasis, Wound Care

Traditional Use:
Kukui nut oil is able to penetrate deep into the skin and scalp and is often used in treatments for dry, damaged skin & hair, to fade scars, to alleviate acne, eczema and psoriasis.

Kukui nut oil is high in Vitamins A, C, E, linoleic acids, and fatty acids and provides anti-oxidants that help to heal and protect the skin making it a traditional topical preparation for treating skin sores, ulcers, and wounds.

Side Effects:
Kukui nut is not recommended for use by women who are pregnant or nursing.

Kukui nut may cause an allergic reaction in some people.

Additional uses and side effects may exist but further research is necessary to determine the exact properties and effects of use.

General:
Kukui nut has been naturalized over nearly every tropical and sub-tropical region of the world. The nut is used as a food, the oils are used as a wood and fiber product varnish and the inner bark yields a dye product used as ink and for cosmetic purposes. The nuts have been used as a body & hair soap.

Kwao Kreu
Botanical Name:
Pueraria mirifica

Common Uses:
Hyper-Pigmentation

Traditional Use:
Kwao Kreu is traditionally used as a topical preparation to reduce hyper-pigmentation like age spots, scarring, and freckles.

Side Effects:
Kwao Kreu is not recommended for use by women who are pregnant or nursing.

Kwao Kreu is not recommended for use by women who have a hormone sensitive condition like endometriosis, fibroids, and certain types of cancers.

Additional uses and side effects may exist but further research is necessary to determine the exact properties and effects of use.

General:
Kwao Kreu is native to Thailand and cultivated in other regions where it has been used as a traditional supplement and commercial supplement.

Labrador Tea
Botanical Name:
Ledum groenlandicum

Common Uses:
Acne, Eczema, Contact Dermatitis, Wound Care

Traditional Use:
Labrador tea leaves have traditionally been used in topical washes & ointments to speed healing and reduce irritation in skin conditions like acne, eczema, and contact dermatitis.

Labrador tea leaves have been included in traditional topical preparations to speed healing in skin sores, ulcers, and wounds.

Part Used:
Leaf

Side Effects:
Labrador Tea is not recommended for use by women who are pregnant or nursing.

Labrador Tea may develop narcotic toxins if allowed to ferment in a closed container for an extended period.

Additional uses and side effects may exist but further research is necessary to determine the exact properties and effects of use.

General:
Labrador tea is made from the leaves of an evergreen shrub found growing naturally in northern climates. The leaves have been used as a refreshing tea, flavoring, and insect repellant.

Lady's Fingers
Kidney Vetch, Lady's Fingers, Woundwort

Botanical Name:
Anthyllis vulneraria

Common Uses:
Acne, Eczema, Wound Care

Traditional Use:
Lady's Fingers have traditionally been used as a wash or ointment in speeding healing and skin regeneration in acne, eczema, skin sores, ulcers, and slow healing wounds.

Part Used:
Leaf, Root

Side Effects:
This is not recommended for use by women who are pregnant or nursing.

Additional uses and side effects may exist but further research is necessary to determine the exact properties and effects of use.

General:
Lady's Fingers are native to Asia and Europe but has been naturalized to North America where it can be found growing wild in grasslands and mountainous regions. The flowers, leaves, and roots are harvested during flowering, dried, and powdered for use in traditional topical preparations.

Lady's Mantle
Lady's Mantle, Lion's Foot, Nine Hooks, Silerkraut, Stellaria

Botanical Name:
Alchemilla vulgaris

Common Uses:
Contact Dermatitis, Wound Care

Traditional Use:
Lady's Mantle has strong astringent, antiseptic, styptic, and vulnerary properties and was considered one of the best herbs for the treatment of bleeding wounds care, for the prevention of infection in burns, and to speed healing in skin sores, ulcers and contact dermatitis.

Part Used:
Root, Whole

Side Effects:
Lady's Mantle is not recommended for use by women who are pregnant or nursing.

Additional uses and side effects may exist but further research is necessary to determine the exact properties and effects of use.

General:
Lady's Mantle is a perennial plant that is indigenous to many regions of the world, growing 10-18 inches in height and blooming in early summer with yellow flowers. It grows easily from seed, cuttings, and division and is a pretty and beneficial component in the garden. The flowers are harvested in the fall and the leaves are harvested during blooming, dried, and powdered for use as a traditional supplement.

Lady's Thumb
Lady's Thumb, Red Leg, Smartweed

Botanical Name:
Polygonum persicaria

Common Uses:
Contact Dermatitis, Wound Care

Traditional Use:
Lady's Thumb has traditionally been used as a topical poultice or wash to alleviate pain and speed healing in skin conditions like sores, ulcers, and wounds.

Part Used:
Bark, Flower, Leaf, Shoot

Side Effects:
Lady's Thumb is not recommended for use by women who are pregnant or nursing.

Lady's Thumb may cause photosensitivity.

Additional uses and side effects may exist but further research is necessary to determine the exact properties and effects of use.

General:
Lady's Thumb is native to Europe but has been naturalized over much of the United States. The flowers, leaves, and shoots are harvested as a cooked or raw vegetable. The bark, flower, leaves, and shoots are all harvested, dried and powdered for use in traditional supplement infusions, extracts, and topical preparations.

Lavender

Botanical Name:
Lavandula angustifolia, Lavendula officinalis

Common Uses:
Acne, Natural Hair & Skin Care

Traditional Use:
Lavender is a core ingredient in many oily skin and acne treatments to help reduce blemishes and kill bacteria. Lavender blends well with astringent carrier oils like grapeseed.

Part Used:
Flower, Leaf, Stem

Side Effects:
Lavender is not recommended for use by women who are pregnant or nursing.

There have been reports that topical use of lavender oil can cause breast growth in boys, men, and young women.

Lavender may cause changes in appetite, constipation, headaches and drowsiness in some people.

Lavender can cause skin irritation in some people.

Lavender is not recommended for use with anti-anxiety, anti-depressants, antihistamines, or sedatives.

Overuse of lavender oil for internal supplements can be toxic if taken by mouth. Oils are for external use only. The leaves can be ingested.

Additional uses and side effects may exist but further research is necessary to determine the exact properties and effects of use.

General:
Lavender is native to the Mediterranean and was used in supplements and ceremonial treatments in ancient Egypt, Greece, and Rome. Lavender is cultivated worldwide for use as a traditional aromatherapy, supplement tea, or extract.

Lemon

Botanical Name:
Citrus limonum

Common Uses:

Acne, Natural Hair & Skin Care

Traditional Use:
Lemon oil helps to brighten dull complexions and is a gentle cleanser for oily skin and hair. The cleansing and antibacterial properties make it a traditional choice for acne treatments. Lemon is also an astringent and is often included in masks to help refresh the skin and prevent the formation of wrinkles.

Lemon oil is traditionally used as a poultice or traditional supplement to strengthen capillaries and help reduce the appearance of varicose veins.

Part Used:
Juice, Rind - Oil

Side Effects:
Lemon is not recommended for use beyond dietary by women who are pregnant or nursing.

Lemon oil is phototoxic oil and should not be used in skin or hair treatments when the user will be exposed to sunlight.

Lemon oil should be diluted when using in any remedy as it may irritate the skin.

Additional uses and side effects may exist but further research is necessary to determine the exact properties and effects of use.

General:
Lemon is native to India but has been cultivated around the world where it is harvested for use in culinary, supplement, cosmetic, and cleaning recipes.

Lemongrass

Citronella, Fever Grass, Lemon Grass, Lemongrass

Botanical Name:
Cymopogon citratus

Common Uses:
Acne, Enlarged Pores, Natural Skin & Hair Care

Traditional Use:
Lemongrass has antibacterial, anti-inflammatory, and astringent properties that make it a traditional ingredient in treating acne and reducing the appearance of large pores.

Lemongrass helps to detoxify the system removing impurities in treatments for acne.

Lemongrass reduces excess oils in skin and hair and is often included in natural shampoos, facial washes, ointments and toners.

Part Used:
Leaf, Stalk, Oil

Side Effects:
Lemon grass is not recommended for use by women who are pregnant or nursing.

Lemon grass may cause an allergic reaction or skin irritation.

Additional uses and side effects may exist but further research is necessary to determine the exact properties and effects of use.

General:
Lemon Grass is native to Asia but is now cultivated in many regions of the world where the stalks are harvested for use as a highly nutritious food and the leaves & oils are harvested and prepared as a traditional supplement tea or essential oil.

Licorice
Black Sugar, Gan-Cao, Licorice, Licorice Root, Sweet Root

Botanical Name:
Glycyrrhiza glabra, Glycyrrhiza uralensis

Common Uses:
Eczema, Psoriasis

Traditional Use:
Licorice is used in topical ointments to sooth skin conditions like eczema, and psoriasis.

Part Used:
Root

Side Effects:
Licorice root containing glycyrrhizin can cause high blood pressure, elevated sodium levels, low potassium levels, and water retention in some people.

Licorice root is not recommended for long-term use.

Licorice is not recommended for use with diuretics, corticosteroids, or other medicines that reduce the body's potassium levels.

Licorice is not recommended for use by women with heart disease or high blood pressure.

Licorice root can affect the body's levels of cortisole.

Licorice root is not recommended for use by women who are pregnant or nursing.

Licorice root might affect estrogen and is not recommended for use by women who have an estrogen related condition.

Licorice root can cause fatigue, headache, menstrual irregularity, water retention and a decrease of sexual function and interest.

Additional uses and side effects may exist but further research is necessary to determine the exact properties and effects of use.

General:
Licorice root is native to Asia, Greece, and Turkey and has a long history of supplement use in both Eastern and Western medicine. Peeled licorice root has traditionally been used in dried, powdered, or extract form. Licorice root sometimes has glycyrrhizin removed that will alter the supplement benefits of the root.

Lime
Botanical Name:
Citrus aurantifolia

Common Uses:
Acne, Natural Skin Care

Traditional Use:
Lime is added to creams to help clear the skin of toxins & oils helping to reduce acne.

Lime is sometimes used as a replacement for lemon in natural hair & skin care recipes.

Part Used:
Oil, Peel

Side Effects:
Lime is not recommended for use beyond dietetic by women who are pregnant or nursing.

Lime oil may cause photosensitivity in some people.

Additional uses and side effects may exist but further research is necessary to determine the exact properties and effects of use.

General:
Lime is native to Asia but is cultivated in other semi-tropic regions where it is harvested for consumption and use in supplements.

Liverwort – Common
Botanical Name:
Marchantia polymorpha

Common Uses:
Eczema

Traditional Use:
Common Liverwort has been used as a traditional topical ointment ingredient to reduce inflammation and speed healing in eczema, skin sores, and skin ulcers.

Part Used:
Leaf

Side Effects:

Common Liverwort is not recommended for use by women who are pregnant or nursing.

Additional uses and side effects may exist but further research is necessary to determine the exact properties and effects of use.

General:
Common Liverwort is found worldwide and prefers moist, tropical zones where the leaves have been harvested, dried, & powdered for use as a traditional supplement. Do not confuse Liverwort Common - Marchantia polymorpha with Liverwort American - Hepatica americana.

Logwood
Bloodwood, Logwood

Botanical Name:
Haematoxylon campechianum

Common Uses:
Skin Pigmentation

Traditional Use:
Logwood is believed to reduce the amount of pigmentation in the skin and is often used in preparations to prevent or reduce freckles, dark scars, and age spots.

Part Used:
Heart Wood

Side Effects:
Logwood is not recommended for use by women who are pregnant or nursing.

Logwood is for external use only. Internal use of Logwood may cause fever, vomiting, and even death in some individuals.

Additional uses and side effects may exist but further research is necessary to determine the exact properties and effects of use.

General:
Logwood is native to North America, Mexico and Central America and is known as the spiny tree. It is used to give grey lavender to blue purple tones in dying or dried and powdered for use in external supplement preparations.

Loosestrife
Blooming Sally, Long Purples, Loosestrife, Purple Loosestrife, Purple Willow Herb, Rainbow Weed, Spiked Loosestrife, Willow Sage

Botanical Name:
Lythrum salicaria

Common Uses:
Eczema, Psoriasis, Wound Care

Traditional Use:
Loosestrife has traditionally been incorporated into internal and external treatments to reduce outbreaks of eczema and psoriasis.

Loosestrife has traditionally been as a topical ointment or wash to prevent infection and speed healing of skin sores, ulcers, and wounds.

Part Used:
Flower, Leaf, Stem

Side Effects:
Loosestrife is not recommended for use by women who are pregnant or nursing.

General:
Loosestrife is a native to Asia, Australia, and North America where the leaves are harvested for use as a calcium rich food, the flowers are used to make culinary colorants, or the flower, leaf, and stem are is harvested while flowering for use fresh or dried. The flower, leave, and stem are traditionally made into infusions for internal use at a rate of up to 3 cups daily and for external washes.

Macadamia Nut
Australian Nut, Bopple Nut, Bush Nut, Macadamia Nut, Queensland Nut

Botanical Name:
Macadamia tetraphylla

Common Uses:
Natural Hair & Skin Care

Carrier Oil

Traditional Uses:
Macadamia Nut oil is an exceptionally light oil and is valued as a carrier oil especially for treatments for those with oily or sensitive skin.

Parts Used:
Nut

Side Effects:
Macadamia Nuts are not recommended for use beyond dietary by women who are pregnant or nursing.

Additional uses and side effects may exist but further research is necessary to determine the exact properties and effects of use.

General:
Macadamia Nuts are native to Australia but are cultivated commercially in other regions where they are harvested for use as a food.

Magnolia

Beaver Tree, Ho No Ki, Holly Bay, Hou Po, Indian Bark, Japanese Whitebark, Magnolia, Red Bay, Red Magnolia, Swamp Laurel, Swamp Sassafras, Sweet Bay, White bay, White Laurel, Xin Ye, Hua

Botanical Name:
Magnolia officinalis

Flower - Analgesic, Anti-Inflammatory, Colorant, Nervine, Sedative

Oil – Antiseptic, Stimulant

Common Uses:
Contact Dermatitis, Hyper-Pigmentation, Wound Care

Traditional Uses:
Magnolia bark and petal oils are traditionally used in topical washes or ointments to reduce itchiness in contact dermatitis and speed healing in skin sores, ulcers, & wounds.

Magnolia has been incorporated into treatments designed to reduce dark skin pigmentation including age spots, freckles, and scarring.

Parts Used:
Bark, Flower Bud

Side Effects:
Magnolia is not recommended for use by women who are pregnant or nursing.

Magnolia may cause heartburn, headaches, sleepiness or tremors.

Additional uses and side effects may exist but further research is necessary to determine the exact properties and effects of use.

General:
Magnolia is a scented ornamental cultivated in many warmer areas of the world. The petals & buds are harvested for use as a food or harvested at the beginning of the flowering season, dried, in the sun, and powdered for use in traditional supplements. The oil is also extracted from the petals by steam distillation for use in aromatherapy and traditional supplements. The bark is harvested for use in an alcohol extraction.

Magnolia – Sweetbay
Laurel Magnolia, Sweetbay Magnolia

Botanical Name:
Magnolia virginiana

Common Uses:
Contact Dermatitis

Traditional Use:

Sweetbay Magnolia has been used as a skin wash to ease discomfort associated with skin sores, skin ulcers, and contact dermatitis like poison ivy.

Part Used:
Bark

Side Effects:
Sweetbay Magnolia is not recommended for use by women who are pregnant or nursing.

Sweetbay Magnolia bark powder may cause dizziness, hallucinations, vision changes or other symptoms.

Additional uses and side effects may exist but further research is necessary to determine the exact properties and effects of use.

General:
Sweetbay Magnolia is a deciduous tree native to the eastern United States where the leaves are harvested, dried and powdered for use as a seasoning and the flower oil is used in perfumery. The bark is harvested, dried, and powdered for use in traditional supplements.

Maidenhair Fern
Five Finger Fern, Maiden Fern, Maidenhair Fern, Rock Fern

Botanical Name:
Adiantum capillus-veneris

Common Uses:
Eczema, Natural Hair Care, Wound Care

Traditional Use:
Maidenhair is traditionally used as a poultice or made into an infusion wash to help reduce the symptoms of eczema and speed healing in skin sores, ulcers, and wounds.

Part Used:
Whole

Side Effects:
Maidenhair is not recommended for use by women who are pregnant or nursing.

Additional uses and side effects may exist but further research is necessary to determine the exact properties and effects of use.

General:
Maidenhair is native along the Atlantic Coast of Europe and North America where it is harvested in the summer, dried, and powdered for use in traditional tea supplements.

Mallow – Common
Common Mallow, High Mallow, Tall Mallow, Malva

Botanical Name:

Malva sylvestris

Common Uses:
Acne, Eczema, Psoriasis, Wound Care

Traditional Use:
Common Mallow has traditionally been used as a topical preparation to sooth inflammation and reduces the appearance of acne.

Common Mallow has traditionally been used as a poultice or ointment to sooth skin inflammation, speed healing and reduce seepage in eczema, psoriasis, sores, ulcers, and wounds.

Part Used:
Leaf

Side Effects:
Common Mallow is not recommended for use by women who are pregnant or nursing.

Common Mallow is not recommended for use by people who have an auto-immune disorder like lupus or multiple sclerosis.

Additional uses and side effects may exist but further research is necessary to determine the exact properties and effects of use.

General:
Common Mallow is native to Africa and Asia but has naturalized to Europe and North America. Common Mallow leaves are eaten as a cooked vegetable. Common Mallow is used as a gentler version of Marsh Mallow and is most commonly used fresh as a decoction.

Mallow – Little
Cheeseweed, Little Mallow

Botanical Name:

Common Uses:
Contact Dermatitis, Eczema, Natural Hair & Skin Care , Psoriasis, Wound Care

Traditional Use:
Little Mallow has been used in natural cosmetic products to soften and smooth the texture of skin and hair and to treat dandruff.

Little Mallow has traditionally been used as a poultice or ointment to sooth skin inflammation, ease pain, speed healing and reduce seepage in contact dermatitis, eczema, psoriasis, sores, ulcers, and wounds.

Part Used:
Leaf, Root, Seed

Side Effects:

Little Mallow is not recommended for use by women who are pregnant or nursing.

Additional uses and side effects may exist but further research is necessary to determine the exact properties and effects of use.

General:
Little Mallow is native to Africa and Asia but is now common to fields & untended areas in most regions of the world. The leaves are harvested for use as a raw or cooked vegetable and the leaves & roots are harvested for use fresh or dried in traditional supplements.

Mallow - Marsh
Althea, Mallards, Marsh Mallow, Marshmallow, Smart Weed, Wymote

Botanical Name:
Althaea officinalis

Common Uses:
Acne, Detoxification, Eczema, Psoriasis

Traditional Use:
Marshmallow root has been used as a traditionally topical preparation to help sooth inflamed skin and speed healing in conditions like acne, eczema, psoriasis, sores, and ulcers.

Marshmallow root has been used as a traditional supplement to bind toxins and detoxify the body in general health treatments and as a supplementary component for conditions like acne, eczema, and psoriasis.

Part Used:
Flower, Root

Side Effects:
Marsh Mallow is not recommended for use by women who are pregnant or nursing.

Marsh Mallow contains high levels of mucilage and pectin that might interfere with the absorption rate of some medications.

Marsh Mallow may lower blood sugar.

Additional uses and side effects may exist but further research is necessary to determine the exact properties and effects of use.

General:
Marsh Mallow is native to Europe but has been naturalized to many regions of the world including North America. Marsh Mallow root is most often used as a food additive. The flowers are harvested during blooming and the root is harvested in the fall for use in traditional supplement teas or tinctures.

Mangosteen

Mangosteen, Queen of Fruits

Botanical Name:
Garcinia mangostana

Common Uses:
Acne

Traditional Uses:
Mangosteen has been used as a traditional supplement to treat certain types of acne by helping to stop the growth of acne causing bacteria.

Parts Used:
Fruit, Heartwood, Leaf, Juice, Rind

Side Effects:
Mangosteen is not recommended for use by women who are pregnant or nursing.

Additional uses and side effects may exist but further research is necessary to determine the exact properties and effects of use.

General:
Mangosteen is a fruit native to the tropical areas of the world where it is harvested as a food but is also used in commercial health drinks & supplements and traditional supplement preparations.

Manketti

Manketti, Mongongo

Botanical Name:
Schinziophyton rautanenii

Common Uses:
Natural Skin Care, Pigmentation – Scarring, Wound Care

Traditional Use:
Manketti oil is hydrating and regenerative and is used in natural skin care products especially for aged skin.

Manketti has traditionally been used in topical treatments to help speed healing in skin sores, ulcers, and wounds while preventing scarring.

Side Effects:
Manketti is not recommended for use by women who are pregnant or nursing.

Additional uses and side effects may exist but further research is necessary to determine the exact properties and effects of use.

General:
Manketti is native to Africa where the nuts are eaten as a food and the oil is harvested by steam distillation for use in cosmetics, aromatherapy, and traditional supplement treatments.

Mares Tail

Common Mare's Tail, Marestail

Botanical Name:
Hippuris vulgaris

Common Uses:
Acne, Wound Care

Traditional Use:
Marestail has been used as a traditional topical preparation to stop bleeding and speed healing in acne, skin sores, skin ulcers, and wounds.

Part Used:
Leaf

Side Effects:
Marestail is not recommended for use by women who are pregnant or nursing.

Additional uses and side effects may exist but further research is necessary to determine the exact properties and effects of use.

General:
Marestail is native to Europe and North America where it can be found growing in bogs & ponds where it is considered an invasive weed by some. The leaves are harvested for use as a fresh or cooked vegetable or used fresh or dried as a traditional supplement.

Masterwort

Botanical Name:
Peucedanum ostruthium

Common Uses:
Contact Dermatitis

Traditional Use:
Masterwort has traditionally been used as a wash or ointment to relieve the itchiness and speed healing of contact dermatitis.

Part Used:
Rhizome, Root

Side Effects:
Masterwort is not recommended for use by women who are pregnant or nursing.

Masterwort may cause photosensitivity in some people.

Additional uses and side effects may exist but further research is necessary to determine the exact properties and effects of use.

General:
Masterwort is native to Europe where the rhizome is harvested in the spring or fall, dried, and powdered for use in traditional infusions up to 3 times daily.

May Chang

May Chang, Tropical Verbena

Botanical Name:
Litsea cubeba

Common Uses:
Acne

Traditional Use:
May Chang has been used as a traditional topical preparation to reduce bacteria and alleviate the severity of acne outbreaks.

Part Used:
Fruit, Oil

Side Effects:
May Chang is not recommended for use by women who are pregnant or nursing.

May Chang is not recommended for internal use by people who have glaucoma or a similar disorder.

May Chang may cause an allergic reaction or skin irritation.

Additional uses and side effects may exist but further research is necessary to determine the exact properties and effects of use.

General:
May Chang is native to Asia and naturalized in other areas where the fruit for use or the oils are extracted by steam distillation for use as a traditional supplement or aromatherapy treatment.

Moneywort

Creeping Jenny, Creeping Joan, Herb Two Pence, Meadow Runagates, Moneywort, Running Jenny, Serpentaria, String of Sovereigns, Twopenny Grass, Wandering Jenny, Wandering Tailor

Botanical Name:
Lysimachia nummularia

Common Uses:
Acne, Eczema, Psoriasis, Wound Care

Traditional Use:
Moneywort has traditionally been used as a wash to ease acne outbreaks.

Moneywort's most common traditional use is as an external wash or ointment component to treat eczema and psoriasis and to help speed wound healing.

Part Used:
Whole

Side Effects:

Moneywort is not recommended for use by women who are pregnant or nursing.

Additional uses and side effects may exist but further research is necessary to determine the exact properties and effects of use.

General:
Moneywort is native to Europe and has been naturalized to North America and Japan where it is harvested while in bloom, dried, and powdered for use in a traditional supplement tea which is taken internally up to 3 times daily or incorporated into a topical preparation.

Mazote

Black Bush, Burweed, Mozote, Sacromento Burbark

Botanical Name:
Triumfetta semitriloba

Common Uses:
Contact Dermatitis, Eczema

Traditional Use:
Mazote has traditionally been used as a topical ointment or to alleviate inflamed, itchy skin conditions like contact dermatitis and eczema.

Part Used:
Leaf

Side Effects:
Mazote is not recommended for use by women who are pregnant or nursing.

Additional uses and side effects may exist but further research is necessary to determine the exact properties and effects of use.

General:
Mazote is native to Central and South America but has become an invasive weed in many tropical regions. The leaves are harvested and used as a tincture or dried and powdered for use in traditional supplement infusions.

Myrrh

Botanical Name:
Commiphora myrrha

Common Uses:
Natural Skin Care, Wound Care

Traditional Use:
Myrrh resin is traditionally used as a topical preparation to speed healing in skin ulcers, cold sores, & canker sores.

Myrrh is believed to have rejuvenating and regenerative effects on the skin making it a common component in natural skin care products especially those designed to reduce scarring.

Part Used:
Resin

Side Effects:
Myrrh is not recommended for use by women who are pregnant or nursing.

Overuse of Myrrh can cause nausea or vomiting.

Myrrh may affect the menstrual cycles in some women.

Individuals with diabetes should consult with a physician before using myrrh as it may affect blood sugar.

Additional uses and side effects may exist but further research is necessary to determine the exact properties and effects of use.

General:
Myrrh is native to the Mediterranean but is cultivated in other regions where the resin is harvested during the summer months for use in perfumery and traditional supplements. The bark is wounded to cause a formation of oily resin that is harvested and the oils extracted by steam distillation.

Neem
Arishtha, Beard Tree, Holy Tree, Indian Lilac, Margosa, Neem

Botanical Name:
Azadirachta Indica

Common Uses:
Acne, Eczema, Natural Hair & Skin Care, Psoriasis, Wound Care

Traditional Use:
Neem leaf tea has been used as a traditional topical preparation to reduce bacterial, inflammation, and dryness associated with acne.

Neem has been used as a traditional topical preparation or soap & shampoo ingredient to relieve the itchiness, redness, and duration of acute eczema and psoriasis outbreaks.

Neem oil has moisturizing and regenerative properties among other components that make it a common ingredient in natural hair, skin, nail, & mouth care cosmetics alleviating conditions like dandruff, dry skin, itchy scalp and hyper pigmentation.

Neem has been used as a traditional topical preparation to reduce infection while speeding healing of skin sores, ulcers, and wounds.

Part Used:

Bark, Leaf, Seed Nut Oil

Side Effects:
Neem is not recommended for use by women who are pregnant or nursing.

Neem is not recommended for use in children's treatments not for internal use.

Neem is not recommended for use by people with an auto-immune disease like Multiple Sclerosis and Lupus.

Neem may lower blood sugar.

Large doses of Neem Oil can be toxic if taken internally – for external use only.

Overuse of Neem may cause diarrhea, drowsiness, loss of consciousness, coma and even death.

Additional uses and side effects may exist but further research is necessary to determine the exact properties and effects of use.

General:
Neem is native to the tropical regions of Africa and Asia where all parts of the tree are harvested. The shoots & flowers of the tree are harvested as a vegetable, the gum is used as a thickening agent, and the stems are used as a tooth cleaning brush. The seeds are harvested and the oil steam extracted or the barks & leaves are harvested, dried, & powdered for use in traditional supplements & cleaning products.

Oak Gall
Botanical Name:
Quercus infectoria

Common Uses:
Skin Infections & Inflammations – Eczema, Psoriasis, Wound

Traditional Use:
Oak Gall bark & seed extract has been used in traditional washes to help heal a variety of skin inflammation and infections including eczema, fissures, frostbite hemorrhoids, psoriasis, skin sores, ulcers, and wounds applied at a rate of 1:5.

Part Used:
Bark, Seed

Side Effects:
Oak Gall is not recommended for use by women who are pregnant or nursing.

Additional uses and side effects may exist but further research is necessary to determine the exact properties and effects of use.

General:

Oak Gall is the Gall produced on the Oak by gall wasps that lay their eggs in the leaf buds of the Oak Tree. The bark & gall are harvested and made into a traditional supplement extract used in topical preparations.

Oats
Avena, Green Oat, Oat, Oatgrass, Oatmeal, Oatstraw, Wild Oat

Botanical Name:
Avena sativa

Common Uses:
Eczema, Psoriasis

Traditional Use:
Oats are traditionally included in poultices and scrubs to sooth the inflammation associated with skin conditions like acne, contact dermatitis, eczema, psoriasis, and sunburns.

Part Used:
Leaf, Stem - Green

Side Effects:
Oats are not recommended for use beyond dietary by women who are pregnant or nursing.

Oats may cause a reaction in individuals who are sensitive to gluten.

Oats may lower blood sugar.

Oats may cause skin irritation in some people.

Additional uses and side effects may exist but further research is necessary to determine the exact properties and effects of use.

General:
Oats are cultivated in much of North America but are also found growing wild in gardens, fields, and elsewhere. Oats are harvested during the flowering season and used fresh in a traditional supplement tea or applied directly or as a tincture to the skin. Processed oats generally have little to no nutritional or supplement value. You should use fresh, green oats whenever attempting to attain the benefits of oat based treatments.

Olive
Acide Gras, Jaitun, Manzanilla Olive, Olive, Olive Leaf, Olive Oil

Botanical Name:
Olea europea

Common Uses:
Natural Hair & Skin Care

Carrier Oil

Traditional Use:
Olive leaf extract has shown to have antioxidant and antimicrobial properties and may be a beneficial component in washes and ointments for disinfecting minor abrasions, cuts, and skin wounds.

Olive oil has long been used as part of natural hair & skin care recipes and is especially effective at treating skin irritation and providing essential nourishment for the hair and skin.

Part Used:
Leaf, Seed Oil

Side Effects:
Olive Oil is not recommended for use beyond dietary by women who are pregnant or nursing.

Olive Oil may cause an allergic reaction in some people.

General:
Olive is cultivated in many regions of the world where the leaves are harvested, shade dried, and used in traditional supplement infusions up to 4 times a day or as oil based dietary or supplement treatment.

Orange - Sweet
Botanical Name:
Citrus sinensis

Common Uses:
Acne, Natural Skin Care

Traditional Use:
Sweet Orange rind has been used as an exfoliating product to alleviate acne.

Part Used:
Oil, Rind

Side Effects:
Sweet Orange is not recommended for use beyond dietary by women who are pregnant or nursing.

Sweet Orange oils may cause increased pigmentation or photosensitivity.

Sweet Orange may cause an allergic reaction or skin irritation.

Additional uses and side effects may exist but further research is necessary to determine the exact properties and effects of use.

General:
Sweet Orange is commonly cultivated as a juice or fruit product, the rind is used as a flavoring and the flowers are cooked as a vegetable or used as a tea product. The rind and oils have been used in cosmetics.

Orange
Botanical Name:
Citrus aurantium

Common Uses:
Natural Skin Care

Traditional Use:
Orange oil is often added to facial and skin care treatments to create a radiant glow and promote fresher, younger looking skin.

Part Used:
Fruit, Rind

Side Effects:
Orange is not recommended for use beyond dietary by women who are pregnant or nursing.

Additional uses and side effects may exist but further research is necessary to determine the exact properties and effects of use.

General:
Orange is commonly cultivated as a juice or fruit product, the rind is used as a flavoring and the flowers are cooked as a vegetable or used as a tea product. The rind and oils have been used in cosmetics, cleaners, and aromatherapy treatments.

Orris Root
Bearded Iris, Daggers, Flag, Flaggon, Flag Lily, Fliggers, Florentine Iris, Gladyne, Iris, Jacob's Sword, Liver Lily, Myrtle Flower, Orris Root, Poison Flag, Purple Flag, Queen Elizabeth Root, Shegg, Snake Lily, Water Flag, White Dragon Flower, Wild Iris, Yellow Flag, Yellow Iris

Botanical Name:
Iris germanica

Common Uses:
Natural Skin Care

Traditional Use:
Orris Root has a pleasant floral scent and is often used as a scent fixative in natural hair & skin care, household cleaning or perfumery products, and perfumes.

Part Used:
Rhizome Root

Side Effects:
Orris is for external use only. Ingestion may cause bloody stools, mouth irritation, stomach pain, and vomiting.

Orris is not recommended for use by women who are pregnant or nursing.

General:
Orris root is naturalized to the United States and can be found growing in a variety of soil, sun, and water

conditions. The root is harvested, dried, and powdered for use in traditional supplements, perfumes, cleaning, and cosmetic products.

Palmarosa
Indian Geranium, Palmarosa

Botanical Name:
Cymbopogon martinii

Common Uses:
Acne, Natural Skin Care, Wound Care

Traditional Use:
Palmarosa oil has antibacterial and astringent properties and is traditionally used to reduce excess oils & bacteria in skin conditions like acne.

Palmarosa oil is used in natural skin care products for its hydrating, regenerative, and balancing effect that leaves the skin supple while aiding in fighting wrinkles.

Palmarosa oil is used in traditional topical preparations to reduce infection and speed healing of skin sores, ulcers, and wounds.

Part Used:
Grass Oils

Side Effects:
Palmarosa oil is not recommended for use by women who are pregnant or nursing.

Palmarosa oil is for external use only.

Additional uses and side effects may exist but further research is necessary to determine the exact properties and effects of use.

General:
Palmarosa is a species of grass related to citronella grass native to Asia and India but cultivated in other regions for its essential oil. The oil is extracted through steam distillation for use in cosmetics, perfumes, and supplements.

Papaya
Melon Tree, Papaya

Botanical Name:
Carica papaya

Common Uses:
Natural Skin Care – Pigmentation, Scar Reduction

Traditional Use:
The milk of the papaya contains high levels of papain and is traditionally used in natural skin care products to remove age spots, freckles, and scarring.

Papaya fruit is traditionally included in poultice

treatments to help reduce scar tissue and has been found to be especially effective in burn care.

Part Used:
Fruit, Leaf

Side Effects:
Papaya is not recommended for use beyond dietary by women who are pregnant or nursing.

Papaya can have a laxative effect.

Papaya leaf, fruit, and seeds contain an anti-parasitic alkaloid that could be dangerous in high doses.

Papaya may cause an allergic reaction or skin irritation.

Additional uses and side effects may exist but further research is necessary to determine the exact properties and effects of use.

General:
Papaya is native to Central and South America where the leaves are harvested early in the growing season and the fruit is harvested when it is ripe.

Patchouli
Huo Xiang, Patchouli, Patchouly, Puthca Pat

Botanical Name:
Pogostermon patchouli

Common Uses:
Acne, Eczema, Natural Skin Care, Skin Scarring, Wound Care

Traditional Use:
Patchouli is used in traditional topical preparations to help treat acne & eczema.

Patchouli is often used in natural skin care recipes for relief from dry, itchy skin and to promote healing.

Patchouli is used as a traditional topical preparation to stimulate cell regeneration, speed healing, and reduce scarring of skin sores, ulcers, and wounds.

Part Used:
Leaf Oil

Side Effects:
Patchouli is not recommended for use by women who are pregnant or nursing.

General:
Patchouli is native to India but can be cultivated worldwide as long as it is protected from frost. The easiest method of propagation is through cuttings. Patchouli Oil is extracted from the leaves for use in topical preparations.

Pea

Common Pea, Garden Pea, Green Pea, Pea

Botanical Name:
Pisum sativum

Common Uses:
Acne

Traditional Use:
Powdered peas have been used as a traditional mask or poultice ingredient to alleviate bacterial skin conditions like acne.

Part Used:
Seed

Side Effects:
Peas are not recommended for use beyond dietary by women who are pregnant or nursing.

Additional uses and side effects may exist but further research is necessary to determine the exact properties and effects of use.

General:
Peas are cultivated in gardens and commercial enterprises as a food product but are also dried & powdered for use as flour or traditional topical preparation or the oils extracted for use as a traditional supplement preparation.

Peach
Botanical Name:
Prunus persica

Common Uses:
Natural Hair & Skin Care

Carrier Oil

Traditional Use:
Peach is used in natural hair & skin care products for its light moisturizing affect suitable for all skin types.

Part Used:
Bark, Leaf, Flower, Fruit, Kernel – Oil

Side Effects:
Peach is not recommended for use beyond dietary by women who are pregnant or nursing.

Additional uses and side effects may exist but further research is necessary to determine the exact properties and effects of use.

General:
Peach trees are native to Asia but have been naturalized in many other regions where the fruit is cultivated as a food.

Peanut
Botanical Name:

Arachis hypogaea

Common Uses:
Eczema, Natural Hair & Skin Care

Traditional Use:
Peanut oil is emollient and antioxidant rich making it a preferred ingredient in natural skin care especially for relief from premature aging and extremely dry skin conditions including eczema, and dandruff reduction.

Part Used:
Seed - Oil

Side Effects:
Peanut is not recommended for use beyond dietary by women who are pregnant or nursing.

Peanut may lower blood pressure.

Peanut may increase bleeding.

Peanut should not be used without the advice of a physician or qualified herbalist.

Additional uses and side effects may exist but further research is necessary to determine the exact properties and effects of use.

General:
Peanuts are cultivated as a food product eaten and have been used as a traditional supplement for thousands of years. The seeds and oil are used in both internal and external supplements and dietary preparations.

Perilla
Perilla, Shiso

Botanical Name:
Perilla frutescens

Common Uses:
Contact Dermatitis, Eczema

Traditional Use:
Perilla has been used as a traditional supplement to alleviate reactive skin conditions like contact dermatitis and eczema.

Part Used:
Leaf, Seed, Stem

Side Effects:
Perilla is not recommended for use by women who are pregnant or nursing.

Additional uses and side effects may exist but further research is necessary to determine the exact properties and effects of use.

General:

Perilla is a perennial herb native to Asia, Europe and North America. It is an easily propagated member of the mint family that spreads by runner and is considered an invasive weed by some. The leaves are harvested for use as a raw or cooked vegetable, the purple leaves are harvested for use as a textile or culinary colorant, and the seed oil is used in making waterproofing products. The leaves, seeds, and stems are harvested, dried, and powdered for use as a traditional supplement.

Petitgrain
Botanical Name:
Petitgrain bigarade

Common Uses:
Acne, Natural Hair & Skin Care

Traditional Use:
Pettigrain is antibacterial and astringent making it a traditional ingredient in acne treatment washes.

Petitgrain oil is used in natural cosmetic products to combat oily skin and hair.

Part Used:
Leaf

Side Effects:
Petitgrain is not recommended for use by women who are pregnant or nursing.

Additional uses and side effects may exist but further research is necessary to determine the exact properties and effects of use.

General:
Petitgrain oil is extracted from the leaves or unripe fruit of the orange tree by steam distillation and is used in perfumery, aromatherapy, and traditional supplements.

Phellodendron
Cork Bark, Cork Tree, Phellodendron

Botanical Name:
Phellodendron amurense

Common Uses:
Eczema, Psoriasis

Traditional Uses:
Phellodendron bark is traditionally included in topical ointments to alleviate the skin symptoms of conditions like eczema and psoriasis.

Parts Used:
Bark

Side Effects:
Phellodendron is not recommended for use by women who are pregnant or nursing.

Phellodendron is not recommended for use in children's treatments.

Phellodendron may lower blood sugar.

Phellodendron is not recommended for use without the guidance of a physician or qualified herbalist.

Additional uses and side effects may exist but further research is necessary to determine the exact properties and effects of use.

General:
Phellodendron is a tree native to Asia and should not be confused with the cultivated houseplant commonly called Philodendron. Phellodendron seeds are harvested for their oil, the wood is used as furniture product, and the bark is used to make cork. The bark is also harvested from mature trees, dried, and powdered for use as a traditional supplement.

Picao Preto
Broomstick, Picao Preto, Spanish Needle

Botanical Name:
Bidens pilosa

Common Uses:
Acne, Wounds

Traditional Use:
Picoa has traditionally been used as a topical preparation to treat bacterial infections like staphylococcus and to combat certain types of acne.

Picoa has been used as a traditional topical wash or ointment to reduce infection, stop bleeding, and speed healing in skin sores, ulcers, and wounds.

Part Used:
Whole

Side Effects:
Picoa is not recommended for use by women who are pregnant or nursing.

Additional uses and side effects may exist but further research is necessary to determine the exact properties and effects of use.

General:
Picao is native to many tropical regions and cultivated in many warmer areas where the shoots & leaves are eaten as a raw or cooked vegetable, or the whole plant is harvested for use as a traditional supplement infusion.

Pipsissewa
Ground Holly, Pipsissewa

Botanical Name:
Chimaphila umbellate

Common Uses:
Acne, Eczema

Traditional Use:
Pipissewa has been used as a traditional supplement to remove toxins from the body and reduce skin conditions like acne & eczema.

Part Used:
Leaf

Side Effects:
Pipsissewa is not recommended for use by women who are pregnant or nursing.

Additional uses and side effects may exist but further research is necessary to determine the exact properties and effects of use.

General:
Pipsissewa is a flowering evergreen native to much of the Northern Hemisphere where the leaves are harvested during the flowering season for use as a flavoring or dried and powdered for use as a traditional supplement.

Pomegranate
Dadima, Pomegranate

Botanical Name:
Punica granatum

Common Uses:
Eczema, Natural Hair & Skin Care, Psoriasis

Traditional Use:
Pomegranate oils are valued for their ability to treat dry skin, eczema, and psoriasis as well as their ability to moisturize and regenerate aging skin while reducing the appearance of fine lines & wrinkles. Some research is being conducted to determine if the tannins and other compounds found in pomegranate oils are of benefit in preventing the formation of UV induced skin cancer.

Part Used:
Bark, Fruit, Oil, Rind, Seed

Side Effects:
Pomegranate is not recommended for use by women who are pregnant or nursing.

Pomegranate bark extracts are very toxic. Do not use bark extracts.

Pomegranate may cause an allergic reaction in some people.

Additional uses and side effects may exist but further research is necessary to determine the exact properties and effects of use.

General:
Pomegranate is native to Africa, China, and India and has been naturalized to parts of California and Arizona easily propagated by seed it is cultivated as an ornamental plant in full sun and well-drained soil.

Pond Lily
Cow Cabbage, Pond Lily, Water Cabbage, Water Lily, White Pond Lily

Botanical Name:
Nymphaea odorata – N alba

Common Uses:
Eczema, Wounds

Traditional Use:
Pond Lily is included in a poultice to treat skin conditions including boils, eczema, and inflamed or infected skin.

Pond Lily is used in traditional topical preparations to speed healing in skin sores, ulcers, and wounds.

Part Used:
Rhizome, Flower - Seed

Side Effects:
Pond Lily is not recommended for use by women who are pregnant or nursing.

Pond Lily may lower blood pressure.

Additional uses and side effects may exist but further research is necessary to determine the exact properties and effects of use.

General:
The White Pond Lily is native to North America and is naturalized throughout the world growing underwater. The rhizome is harvested in the autumn, dried, and powdered for use in external wash, poultice, or ointment preparations of 1 part powder to 1 part ethanol or ¼ teaspoon powder to 1 teaspoon liquid base daily. For acute conditions of the throat 5 drops of the external tincture is traditionally given up to 3 times daily.

Prickly Ash
Hercules Club, Pepper Wood, Prickly Ash, Toothache Bark, Yellow Wood

Botanical Name:
Zanthoxylum rhetsa

Common Uses:
Contact Dermatitis, Eczema

Traditional Use:
Prickly Ash bark has been used as a traditional topical preparation to alleviate skin irritation and itching

associated with conditions like contact dermatitis and eczema.

Part Used:
Bark

Side Effects:
Prickly Ash is not recommended for use by women who are pregnant or nursing.

Prickly Ash is not recommended for use by people who have intestinal conditions like IBS or Crohn's disease.

Additional uses and side effects may exist but further research is necessary to determine the exact properties and effects of use.

General:
Prickly Ash is a deciduous shrub where it can be found growing along the coastlines. The seeds are harvested for use as a culinary spice and the pods are used as a natural colorant. The bark, fruit, and root are all harvested for use as traditional medicinals but the root is most frequently used.

Psyllium
Botanical Name:
Plantago psyllium

Common Uses:
Natural Hair & Skin Care

Traditional Use:
Plantago psyllium seeds are a good source of fiber and can absorb up to 14 times its weight in water making it a useful thickening agent in natural skin and hair care products.

Part Used:
Seed, Seed Husks

Side Effects:
Psyllium is not recommended for use by women who are pregnant or nursing.

Psyllium seeds should not be used with any other stimulant laxative.

Psyllium seeds may interfere with the absorption of essential minerals, nutrients, vitamins, and medications and is not for long term use.

Drink plenty of fluids whenever Psyllium is being used as a dietary or supplement component.

Additional uses and side effects may exist but further research is necessary to determine the exact properties and effects of use.

General:
Psyllium Seeds come from the Plantain plant native to many countries of the world and can be found growing

wild in much of North America. The seeds are harvested for use as a cosmetic, dietary, or medicinal product.

Pumpkin Seed
Calabaza, Curcurbita, Pumpkin, Pumpkin Seed

Botanical Name:
Cucurbita pepo

Common Uses:
Natural Hair & Skin Care

Traditional Use:
Pumpkin seed oil is beneficial in healing dry, damaged skin including skin suffering from minor abrasions, cuts, and wounds.

Part Used:
Oil, Seed

Side Effects:
Pumpkin seeds & oil are not recommended for use women who are pregnant or nursing.

Pumpkin seed & oil may affect a developing fetus.

Pumpkin and Pumpkin Seed may cause indigestion and diarrhea in some individuals.

Additional uses and side effects may exist but further research is necessary to determine the exact properties and effects of use.

General:
Pumpkin seed is often dried and powdered and seed oil should be cold pressed and consumed uncooked as heat can minimize the beneficial properties.

Rabbitbrush
Botanical Name:
Ericameria nauseosa

Common Uses:
Acne, Wound Care

Traditional Use:
Rabbitbrush has been used in traditional topical preparations to reduce skin inflammations like acne and to speed healing of skin sores, ulcers, and wounds.

Part Used:
Stems, Twigs

Side Effects:
Rabbitbrush is not recommended for use by women who are pregnant or nursing.

Rabbitbrush is not recommended for internal use without the advice of a physician or qualified herbalist.

Overuse of Rabbitbrush may cause an extreme drop in blood pressure.

Additional uses and side effects may exist but further research is necessary to determine the exact properties and effects of use.

General:
Rabbitbrush is a shrub native to North America where it is cultivated as an ornamental or as a forage plant. The leaves have been used as a sanitary padding, the flower head as a stuffing material, and the root sap as a source of hypoallergenic rubber or gum product.

Radish
Botanical Name:
Raphanus sativus

Common Uses:
Acne, Natural Skin Care

Traditional Use:
Radish is traditionally used in topical preparations to remove excess oils related to oily skin and reduce the severity of certain types of acne outbreaks.

Part Used:
Leaf, Root, Seed

Side Effects:
Radish is not recommended for use beyond dietary by women who are pregnant or nursing.

Additional uses and side effects may exist but further research is necessary to determine the exact properties and effects of use.

General:
Radish is cultivated as a food source worldwide and is also harvested for traditional supplement use with 1 radish grated to a juice pulp and mixed in a base, steeped for 12-24 hours and used at a rate of 1 spoonful every hour until symptoms abate.

Ragweed
Giant Ragweed, Horseweed, Ragweed

Botanical Name:
Ambrosia trifida

Common Uses:
Acne, Contact Dermatitis

Traditional Use:
Ragweed leaf juices have been used in traditional topical preparations to treat bacterial infections and to reduce the severity of acne outbreaks.

Crushed Ragweed have been used as a topical preparation to alleviate the inflammation, itchiness, and seepage associated with conditions like insect bites, stings, and contact dermatitis like poison ivy.

Part Used:
Flower, Leaf

Side Effects:
Ragweed is not recommended for use by women who are pregnant or nursing.

Ragweed can cause severe allergic reactions in some people.

Additional uses and side effects may exist but further research is necessary to determine the exact properties and effects of use.

General:
Ragweed is considered a weed found growing throughout untended areas of North America but it was cultivated by the Native Americans as an oil producing plant and food product.

Raspberry
Framboise, Raspberry, Raspberry Leaf

Botanical Name:
Rubus idaeus

Common Uses:
Acne, Natural Hair & Skin Care, Wound Care

Traditional Use:
Raspberry leaves have shown an astringent and local anti-inflammatory effect making it a traditional ingredient for poultices, masks, and washes for the treatment of acne, hemorrhoids, and skin wounds.

Raspberry leaf has been used in traditional topical preparations to speed healing in skin sores, ulcers, and wounds.

Part Used:
Bark, Fruit, Leaf

Side Effects:
Raspberry Leaf Tea is not recommended for use by women who are pregnant or nursing.

Raspberry Leaf Tea is not recommended for use by women who have a hormone sensitive condition like endometriosis, fibroids or certain types of cancer.

Raspberry leaf may cause uterine contractions.

Use fully dried leafs as the leaf develops toxins during the drying process that can cause nausea in some people.

Additional uses and side effects may exist but further research is necessary to determine the exact properties and effects of use.

General:

Raspberry can be found in many regions of the world and is native to much of North America and Canada. Though raspberry can thrive in a variety of conditions, it does prefer partly shaded areas for optimal growth. The fruit is harvested as a food and the leaves are harvested, dried, powdered and incorporated into traditional supplement teas.

Ravensara
Botanical Name:
Ravensara Aromatica

Common Uses:
Acne, Wound Care

Traditional Use:
Ravensara has been used as a traditional topical preparation to reduce the severity of acne outbreaks and to treat bacterial infections.

Ravensara is used in traditional preparations to reduce the likelihood of infections in skin wounds.

Part Used:
Bark – Leaf – Oil

Side Effects:
Ravensara is not recommended for use by women who are pregnant or nursing.

Additional uses and side effects may exist but further research is necessary to determine the exact properties and effects of use.

General:
Ravensara is native to Madagascar and cultivated elsewhere for the essential oils extracted from the bark & leaves. The oils are extracted through steam distillation and used in topical and aromatherapy preparations.

Red Clover
Beebread, Cloveone, Cow Clover, Daidzein, Meadow Clover, Purple Clover, Red Clover, Wild Clover

Botanical Name:
Trifolium pratense

Common Uses:
Acne, Eczema, Psoriasis

Traditional Use:
Red clover has traditionally been used as an external wash for relief from skin conditions like acne, eczema, and psoriasis.

Red Clover tea is given up to 3 times daily as a traditional supplement to help purify the blood in treatment plans for acne, arthritis, and gout.

Part Used:
Flower

Side Effects:
Red clover is not recommended for use by women who are pregnant or nursing.

Red clover is not recommended for use by women who have a hormone sensitive condition like endometriosis, fibroids, or certain types of cancer.

Red clover is not recommended for use by people with a bleeding disorder.

Red clover may have contraceptive effects by rendering the cervix less accessible to sperm entry and should not be used by anyone attempting to conceive.

Red clover may cause an allergic reaction or skin irritation.

Additional uses and side effects may exist but further research is necessary to determine the exact properties and effects of use.

General:
The flowers of the Red Clover are found in many regions of the world including Asia, Africa, Europe, North America, and South America. The leaves and flowering tops have been used in traditional supplement teas, tinctures, extracts, and powders. Red clover belongs to the legume family and is native to North America and can be found growing wild in open meadows and fields.

Reed - Common
Ditch Reed, Giant Reed, Reed

Botanical Name:
Phragmites australis

Common Uses:
Contact Dermatitis, Wound Care

Traditional Use:
Reed juice is traditionally included in topical applications to relieve the itchiness and inflammation of contact dermatitis and insect bites.

Reed leaves have traditionally been burnt to ashes and used as a poultice to help speed healing in seeping sores, ulcers, and wounds.

Part Used:
Rhizome, Stem

Side Effects:
Reed is not recommended for use by women who are pregnant or nursing.

Reed resin smoke may cause psychoactive effects and caution should be employed when burning fresh reeds.

Additional uses and side effects may exist but further research is necessary to determine the exact properties and effects of use.

General:
The Common Reed is a perennial grass that can be found in tropical or semi-tropical regions growing in wetlands. The reeds have been harvested for use in basket making, thatching, to make brooms, musical instruments or weaponry. The young stems have been harvested, dried & powdered for use as a flour product or roasted as a whole food. The whole plant has been fermented for use as a cleaning and fuel alcohol. The root is harvested in the fall, juiced or powdered for inclusion in traditional supplements.

Rooibos
Green Bush Tea, Kaffree Tea, Red Tea, Red Bush Tea, Rooibos

Botanical Name:
Aspalathus linearis

Common Uses:
Acne, Eczema, Psoriasis

Traditional Use:
The anti-histamine ability of Rooibos has made it a traditional ingredient in teas to minimize reactive conditions like acne, asthma, eczema, psoriasis, and seasonal allergies.

Part Used:
Branch, Leaf

Side Effects:
Rooibos is not recommended for use by women who are pregnant or nursing.

Additional uses and side effects may exist but further research is necessary to determine the exact properties and effects of use.

General:
Rooibos is native to Africa where it is harvested, chopped, and allowed to sun dry for use as a tea. Rooibos should be slow dried using only natural lighting. The tea is used as a traditional supplement.

Rose
Botanical Name:
Rosa centifolia

Common Uses:
Acne, Natural Skin Care – Inflammation, Wound Care

Traditional Use:
Rose petals and bark are used to make an astringent skin care wash that is traditionally used to reduce acne outbreaks, disinfect minor wounds, and speed the healing process of damaged skin.

Rose water is often used as a facial toning ingredient and has anti-inflammatory compounds that may make it beneficial in treating skin inflammations including mild acne.

Part Used:
Bark, Flower - Oil

Side Effects:
Rose is not recommended for use by women who are pregnant or nursing.

Additional uses and side effects may exist but further research is necessary to determine the exact properties and effects of use.

General:
Roses are cultivated as an aromatic ornamental in most regions of the world. The highest supplement qualities can be found in non-hybrid roses whose tea and oils are a deep red tone.

Rosebay
Rhododendron, Rosebay, Snow Rose

Botanical Name:
Rhododendron aureum

Common Uses:
Acne, Bacterial Infections, Wound Care

Traditional Use:
Rosebay oil has traditionally been used as a topical ointment to alleviate certain types of acne.

Part Used:
Flower, Leaf, Stem

Side Effects:
Rosebay is not recommended for use by women who are pregnant or nursing.

Internal use of Rosebay may cause inebriation and is considered toxic.

Additional uses and side effects may exist but further research is necessary to determine the exact properties and effects of use.

General:
Rosebay is a shrub native to Asia & Europe and cultivated in mountainous regions where the flowers are harvested during flowering & dried for use as a traditional supplement while the flowers, leaves, and stems are harvested and the oils extracted through steam distillation for use in topical preparations

Rose – Eglantine
Rose – Eglantine, Sweet Briar

Botanical Name:
Rosa rubiginosa

Common Uses:
Natural Skin Care – Anti-Aging, Scar Reduction, Wound Care

Traditional Use:
Eglantine Rose petals are traditionally used to speed healing of skin sores, skin ulcers, and minor wounds.

Eglantine Rose seed oils are rich in vitamin E and have been used in natural skin care products to reduce the signs of aging, the appearance of scars and to speed healing of minor skin wounds.

Part Used:
Flower, Fruit, Seed – Oil

Side Effects:
Eglantine Rose is not recommended for use by women who are pregnant or nursing.

Eglantine Rose may cause mouth, throat, or gastro-intestinal irritation.

Additional uses and side effects may exist but further research is necessary to determine the exact properties and effects of use.

General:
Eglantine Rose is traditionally cultivated as an ornamental or hedge shrub. The fruit is harvested for use as a cooked jelly or vitamin rich tea product. The petals and shoots are eaten as a raw or cooked vegetable. The seeds have been ground into powder and used as a flour nutritional supplement. Oils are steam extracted from the fruits & seeds for use in topical and supplement products.

Rose Geranium
Botanical Name:
Pelargonium odorantissimum

Common Uses:
Acne, Natural Skin Care

Traditional Uses:
Rose Geranium is a has a light citrus-rose scent that makes it a common ingredient in perfumed cosmetics and is traditionally used to help clear the skin of excess oil while promoting healing making it a common ingredient in skin care recipes for oily and acne prone skin.

Parts Used:
Leaf, Stem

Side Effects:
Rose Geranium is not recommended for use by women who are pregnant or nursing.

Rose Geranium may cause skin irritation.

Additional uses and side effects may exist but further research is necessary to determine the exact properties and effects of use.

General:
Rose Geranium is native to Africa and Egypt but is cultivated in many regions where the leaves are harvested at the end of the season and the oils extracted for use in perfumes and traditional medicinals.

Rose Hip
Common Uses:
Anti-Aging, Natural Skin Care

Traditional Uses:
Rose hip oils are naturally high in GLA, contain collagen stimulating compounds, and help to reduce fine lines and wrinkles while preventing scarring making them a common ingredient in natural skin & wound care products.

Parts Used:
Hip, Seed

Side Effects:
Rose Hips are not recommended for use by women who are pregnant or nursing.

Rosehips may affect blood sugar.

Overuse of rose hips may cause diarrhea, fatigue, heartburn, nausea, sleep interruption, and vomiting.

Rosehip oil may aggravate acne in some people.

Additional uses and side effects may exist but further research is necessary to determine the exact properties and effects of use.

General:
The rose hips are the rounded portion of the flower just below the petals and contain the seeds of the rose. The rose hip is dried, powdered and used in traditional supplement infusions or the oil is extracted by steam distillation for use in topical, aromatherapy, or traditional supplements.

Rosewood
Bois de Rosa, Rosewood

Botanical Name:
Aniba rosaeodora

Common Uses:
Natural Skin Care

Traditional Use:
Rosewood oil regenerates damaged skin while infusing moisture and is a beneficial component in many skin care treatments including creams, lotions, massage treatments, and soaps with an added benefit of a beautiful scent.

Part Used:
Bark – Oils

Side Effects:
Rosewood is not recommended for use by women who are pregnant or nursing.

Additional uses and side effects may exist but further research is necessary to determine the exact properties and effects of use.

General:
Rosewood is a tree native to the Amazon where the wood is harvested for use in furniture making and the oils extracted through steam distillation for use in perfumery, aromatherapy, and as a traditional supplement.

Safflower
Alazor, American Saffron, Bastard Saffron, Benibana, Dyer's Saffron, Safflower, Zaffer, Zafran

Botanical Name:
Carthamus tinctorius

Common Uses:
Natural Hair & Skin Care, Psoriasis, Wound Care

Traditional Use:
Safflower oil is highly moisturizing and is frequently used as a base or component in natural hair and skin care products designed to treat exceptionally dry or damaged skin.

Safflower petal tea is traditionally used to discourage cell proliferation in treatments for discouraging the excess growth related to conditions like psoriasis.

Safflower petals have traditionally been used to help speed healing and reduce infection in skin sores, ulcers, and wounds.

Part Used:
Flower, Oil

Side Effects:
Safflower has been used as an abortifacient in traditional supplements and should not be used by pregnant or nursing women.

Safflower can increase bleeding and slow clotting.

Safflower may cause an allergic reaction in some people.

Additional uses and side effects may exist but further research is necessary to determine the exact properties and effects of use.

General:
Safflower is native to India, Africa, Europe and North America but is cultivated elsewhere. Safflower is harvested after blooming and dried in the shade, and powdered for use in traditional supplement teas up to 3 times daily. Safflower oil should be used cold in culinary, skin care, and supplement products since heat may diminish the beneficial components of the oil.

Sage Bush – Grey
Grey Sage Bush, Saltbush

Botanical Name:
Atriplex canescens

Common Uses:
Contact Dermatitis, Skin Irritation, Skin Rashes

Traditional Use:
The leaves of the Grey Sage Bush are traditionally used as a soapy skin wash to reduce the pain, inflammation and itchiness of skin irritation, contact dermatitis and other rashes.

Part Used:
Leaf

Side Effects:
Grey Sage Brush is not recommended for use by women who are pregnant or nursing.

Additional uses and side effects may exist but further research is necessary to determine the exact properties and effects of use.

General:
Grey Sage Bush is native to Central America and the southwestern portion of North America where the leaves are harvested for use as a raw or cooked vegetable; the seed is eaten as a cooked snack food or ground into a baking soda substance. The leaves are used as a soap replacement or in traditional topical preparations.

Sandalwood
Anaditam, Chandran, Chandana, Safed Chandan, Sandal Tree, Sandalwood, Santal, Tan Xiang, White Sandalwood, Yellow Sandalwood, Yellow Saunders

Botanical Name:
Santalum album

Common Uses:
Acne, Natural Hair & Skin Care

Traditional Use:
Sandalwood is used as a toning astringent cleanser in natural hair & skin care products especially those designed to treat acne, skin inflammation, and dehydrated skin.

Part Used:

Wood   - Oil

Side Effects:
Sandalwood is not recommended for use other than aromatic by women who are pregnant or nursing.

Overuse of Sandalwood Oil may affect the kidneys.

Sandalwood may cause an allergic reaction to sandalwood including gastrointestinal upset, itching, and nausea.

Additional uses and side effects may exist but further research is necessary to determine the exact properties and effects of use.

General:
Sandalwood oil is extracted from the inner wood of the sandalwood tree. Sandalwood is a semi-parasitic tree that depends on other trees for nourishment early in its development. Sandalwood has been over harvested and presently considered an endangered botanical species. The oils are extracted through steam distillation for use in perfumery, aromatherapy, and supplemental treatments.

Sand Sedge
German Sarsaparilla, Sand Sedge

Botanical Name:
Carex arenaria

Common Uses:
Eczema, Skin Irritation

Traditional Use:
Sand Sedge has been used in topical preparations to reduce the dryness and itchiness associated with conditions like eczema and other skin irritation.

Part Used:
Root

Side Effects:
Sand Sedge is not recommended for use by women who are pregnant or nursing.

Sand Sedge is not recommended for use in children's treatments.

Sand Sedge is not recommended for use by people with sensitivity to aspirin, who have a bleeding disorder or who are on a blood thinning medication.

Additional uses and side effects may exist but further research is necessary to determine the exact properties and effects of use.

General:
Sand Sedge is a perennial ground plant native to Asia, Europe, and North America where it can be found growing wild in sandy areas including sea shores. The

root is harvested, dried, and powdered for use in traditional supplement infusions or made into an alcohol tincture.

Sarsaparilla
Sarsaparilla, Smilax, Zarzaparilla

Botanical Name:
Smilax sarsaparilla

Common Uses:
Acne, Eczema, Natural Hair & Skin Care, PMS, Psoriasis

Traditional Use:
Sarsaparilla has anti-inflammatory and antibacterial properties that may make it a traditional skin wash treatment for certain types of acne, eczema, and psoriasis.

Sarsaparilla has traditionally been used to detoxify the body and reduce impurity related flare ups of conditions like acne, eczema, and psoriasis.

The phytochemicals in Sarsaparilla are believed to help sooth certain inflammatory conditions like acne, eczema, gout, and psoriasis by disabling certain bacterial components that build up in the blood and cause flare ups in each condition.

Sarsaparilla is sometimes used as an emulsifier in natural hair and skin care products.

Part Used:
Root

Side Effects:
Sarsaparilla is not recommended for use by women who are pregnant or nursing.

Sarsaparilla may cause asthma like symptoms in some people.

Over use or overdose of Sarsaparilla can cause kidney damage.

Additional uses and side effects may exist but further research is necessary to determine the exact properties and effects of use.

General:
Sarsaparilla is a woody climbing vine native to China, Central America & South America but cultivated in other regions. Sarsaparilla prefers rich, moist soil and part shade for optimal growth. Sarsaparilla is harvested in the late winter or early spring, dried and powdered for use in traditional supplements up to 3 times daily.

Sea Buckthorn
Common Names:
Argasse, Argousier, Chharma, Dhar Bu, Finbar, Grisset, Meerdorn, Oblepikha, Purging Thorn, Saddorn, Sea Buckthorn, Seedom, Star Bu, Tindved, Yellow Spine

Botanical Name:
Hippophae rhamnoides

Common Uses:
Acne, Anti-Aging, Damaged Skin, Eczema, Natural Skin Care, Seborrhea, Wounds

Traditional Use:
Sea buckthorn berry juice is rich in vitamins, phytosterols, anti-oxidants, and carotenoids. These give the oil potentially regenerative properties making it a traditional treatment for a variety of skin disorders including acne, acute dryness, burns, eczema, and sun damage.

Sea buckthorn is used in natural skin care products to combat the formation of wrinkles and reverse premature aging of the skin caused by exposure to harsh environmental factors.

Sea Buckthorn oils have traditionally been used in topical preparations to speed healing in skin sores, ulcers, and wounds.

Part Used:
Berry, Juice, Seed, Oil

Side Effects:
Sea Buckthorn is not recommended for use by women who are pregnant or nursing.

Sea Buckthorn may reduce blood clotting action and is not recommended for use by people on blood thinning supplements, with a blood clotting disorder or who are undergoing surgery.

Undiluted sea buckthorn oil may stain the skin and other items.

Additional uses and side effects may exist but further research is necessary to determine the exact properties and effects of use.

General:
Sea Buckthorn is a hardy shrub native to China and Russia and grows naturally along the sea shore but can also be found in other habitats and regions. Sea Buckthorn is available in concentrates, juices, oils or powdered form and the traditional daily dosage is 10 grams.

Sea Grape
Bay Grape, Sea Grape

Botanical Name:
Coccoloba uvifera

Common Uses:
Acne, Wound Care

Traditional Use:

Sea Grape has been used as a traditional topical wash to help alleviate the severity of acne outbreaks.

Sea Grape has been used as a traditional topical preparation to speed healing and reduce the likelihood of infection in skin sores, ulcers, and wounds.

Part Used:
Bark – Gum, Leaf,

Side Effects:
Sea Grape is not recommended for use by women who are pregnant or nursing.

Sea Grape lowers blood sugar and should not be used without the advice of a physician or qualified herbalist.

Additional uses and side effects may exist but further research is necessary to determine the exact properties and effects of use.

General:
Sea Grape is a small tree native to the shoreline in Central America, South America and North America. The fruit is harvested for use as a cooked fruit and the bark, leaf, and fruit is harvested for use in supplement or topical decoctions.

Sesame
Botanical Name:
Sesamum indicum

Common Uses:
Natural Hair & Skin Care

Traditional Use:
Sesame seed oil is rich in vitamins A & E and contains essential proteins and anti-oxidants making it a frequently used carrier oil for natural hair & skin care products.

Part Used:
Seed, Seed Oil

Side Effects:
Sesame Seed is not recommended for use by women who are pregnant or nursing.

Additional uses and side effects may exist but further research is necessary to determine the exact properties and effects of use.

General:
Sesame is native to Africa and India but is naturalized to many tropical regions and is cultivated worldwide as a culinary seasoning, cooking oil, cosmetic ingredient, supplement or natural hair & skin care product ingredient.

Shatavari
Shatavari, Sathavari, Thaneevittan

Botanical Name:
Asparagus racemosus

Common Uses:
Acne

Traditional Use:
Shatavari has been used in topical washes to prevent certain types of bacterial acne and as a supplement to prevent hormonally stimulated acne outbreaks.

Part Used:
Whole

Side Effects:
Shatavari is not recommended for use by women who are pregnant or nursing.

Additional uses and side effects may exist but further research is necessary to determine the exact properties and effects of use.

General:
Shatavari is a species of asparagus native to India and cultivated in other regions where it is harvested for use as a food or for use as a traditional supplement treatment.

Shea Nut
Shea Nut, Shea Butter

Botanical Name:
Butyrospermum parkii

Common Uses:
Eczema, Natural Hair & Skin Care, Skin Irritation & Rashes

Traditional Use:
Shea butter is an intense moisturizer and is rich in vitamins, minerals and natural humectants that help to hydrate hair & skin. Shea Butter also helps to protect the skin from free radicals and may help to combat the formation of fine lines & wrinkles making it a common ingredient in skin & hair care products.

Shea butter is traditionally used to sooth skin irritation and infuses moisture while speeding healing in conditions like eczema.

Part Used:
Nuts

Side Effects:
Additional uses and side effects may exist but further research is necessary to determine the exact properties and effects of use.

General:
Shea trees are native to Africa where the nuts are harvested as a food plant, chocolate making product, and as a traditional cosmetic and supplement product.

Silverweed

Botanical Name:
Potentilla anserina

Common Uses:
Contact Dermatitis, Natural Skin Care

Protection

Traditional Use:
Silverweed is used in traditional topical preparations to reduce discomfort associated with contact dermatitis like poison ivy.

Silverweed has traditionally been used as a soothing skin wash and is sometimes included in natural skin care cleaning products.

Part Used:
Root, Stem

Side Effects:
Silverweed is not recommended for use by women who are pregnant or nursing.

Additional uses and side effects may exist but further research is necessary to determine the exact properties and effects of use.

General:
Silverweed is a flowering perennial native throughout the northern hemisphere where it can be found growing wild along rivers, roadsides, and forest edges. The roots have been harvested for use as a raw or cooked vegetable or dried & powdered for use as a thickening agent or flour. The leaves and roots are harvested in the summer, dried, and powdered for use in traditional topical and supplement treatments.

Skullcap

Blue Pimpernel, Helmet Flower, Hoodwort, Mad Dog Weed, Quaker Bonnet, Skullcap

Botanical Name:
Scutellaria lateriflora

Common Uses:
Contact Dermatitis

Traditional Use:
Skullcap is traditionally added as a component in skin washes and ointments for rashes resulting from allergic reactions to environmental irritants.

Part Used:
Flower, Leaf, Stem

Side Effects:
Skullcap is not recommended for use by women who are pregnant or nursing.

Overuse or overdose can cause confusion, hallucinations, and seizures.

Skullcap may have a sedative effect and you should not drive or operate heavy machinery while using skullcap.

Ensure you use only skullcap that contains scutellarin as other species of skullcap do not have the same compounds.

Additional uses and side effects may exist but further research is necessary to determine the exact properties and effects of use.

General:
Skullcap is found throughout the United States and prefers shaded areas with moist soil. It is harvested, dried, and powdered for use in traditional powder and extract supplements.

Snowberry

Botanical Name:
Symphoricarpos albus laevigatus

Common Uses:
Contact Dermatitis, Wound Care

Traditional Use:
Snowberry bark, leaves, & roots have traditionally been used in poultice and wash preparations to speed healing in skin sores, ulcers, and wounds.

Snowberry fruit have been used as a topical wash or mashed as a poultice to remove warts.

Part Used:
Bark, Fruit, Leaf

Side Effects:
Snowberry is not recommended for use by women who are pregnant or nursing.

Snowberry is not recommended for internal use without the advice of a physician or qualified herbalist.

Additional uses and side effects may exist but further research is necessary to determine the exact properties and effects of use.

General:
Snowberry is native to Asia, Central America and North America where it was commonly used as a topical medicinal by the Native Americans. The berries have been harvested for use as a soap alternative and the bark, fruit, and leaves have been used in topical preparations.

Soapwort

Bouncing Bet, Bruisewort, Fullers Herb, Red Soapwort

Botanical Name:

Saponaria officinalis

Common Uses:
Eczema, Natural Hair & Skin Care, Psoriasis

Traditional Use:
Soapwort is a common ingredient in cleaning products and skin care cleansers. Soapwort creates a mild lather on contact with water and leaves behind a silky, slippery feeling.

Soapwort has traditionally been used as a topical preparation in the treatment of chronic skin conditions including eczema and psoriasis.

Part Used:
Leaf, Rhizome

Side Effects:
Soapwort is not recommended for use by women who are pregnant or nursing.

Soapwort is not recommended for use by people with inflammatory bowel disease or ulcers.

Soapwort is a purgative that may cause nausea, stomach irritation, and vomiting.

Soapwort is not recommended for internal use without the advice of a physician or qualified herbalist.

Soapwort may irritate the skin or mucus membranes.

Additional uses and side effects may exist but further research is necessary to determine the exact properties and effects of use.

General:
Soapwort is native to Asia, Europe and North America and can be found growing wild along roadsides and untended areas where the roots and leaves are harvested during the flowering season and used fresh or dried for use in traditional supplement teas or decoctions.

Sour Cherry
Albulak, Alubalu, Pie Cherry, Sour Cherry

Botanical Name:
Prunus cerasus

Common Uses:
Aging

Traditional Uses:
Sour Cherry contains powerful anti-oxidants and has been used as a traditional supplement to slow the aging process, repair cell damage, and support brain & body health.

Parts Used:
Fruit, Juice

Side Effects:
Sour Cherry is not recommended for use beyond dietary by women who are pregnant or nursing.

Additional uses and side effects may exist but further research is necessary to determine the exact properties and effects of use.

General:
Sour Cherry is a species of cherry native to Asia and Europe and naturalized to the United States where it is cultivated as an ornamental. The fruits are harvested for use as a food flavoring, cooked or raw fruit, and in traditional supplements.

Spearmint
Curled Mint, Fresh Mint, Garden Mint, Green Mint, Lamb Mint, Mackerel Mint, Our Lady's Mint, Pahari Pudina, Sage of Bethlehem, Spearmint, Spire Mint, Yerba Buena

Botanical Name:
Mentha spicata

Common Uses:
Natural Skin Care

Traditional Use:
Spearmint is used in facial steam treatments and toning washes to cleanse & tighten pores.

Part Used:
Leaf, Oil

Side Effects:
Spearmint is not recommended for use by women who are pregnant or nursing.

General:
Spearmint is found in nearly every country of the world and is adapted to a variety of soil, sun, and water conditions. It is considered an invasive weed by some. Spearmint oil is extracted from the flower, leaf, and stem harvested during the flowering season.

Speedwell
Gypsy weed, Speedwell, Veronica

Botanical Name:
Veronica officinalis

Common Uses:
Eczema, Psoriasis, Skin Irritation & Rash

Traditional Use:
Speedwell tea is traditionally used as a soothing wash to speed wound healing, calm itchy or irritated skin, and in treatments for eczema and psoriasis.

Part Used:
Flower, Leaf, Stem

Side Effects:
Speedwell is not recommended for use by women who are pregnant or nursing.

General:
Speedwell is native to Asia, Europe, and North America, Europe, and Asia and can be found growing in fields, ponds, and untended areas where it is harvested during the flowering season, dried, and powdered for use in traditional teas that have been given up to 3 times daily and externally as needed for relief from symptoms.

Spikenard
Fleabane, Indian Root, Old Man's Root, Pettymorell, Spignet, Spikenard

Botanical Name:
Aralia racemosa

Common Uses:
Contact Dermatitis, Natural Skin Care

Traditional Use:
Spikenard has been used as a traditional topical preparation to reduce inflammation and discomfort associated with skin conditions like contact dermatitis.

Spikenard is used in natural skin care products for its rejuvenating anti-inflammatory effects and is especially prized in treatments for mature skin.

Part Used:
Root

Side Effects:
Spikenard is not recommended for use by women who are pregnant or nursing.

Spikenard may cause skin irritation.

Additional uses and side effects may exist but further research is necessary to determine the exact properties and effects of use.

General:
Spikenard is native to the United States and can be found growing wild in open woods, thickets, and untended areas where it is harvested, dried, and powdered for use in traditional supplement infusions up to 3 times daily.

Stonecrop
Bird Bread, Biting Stonecrop, Creeping Tom, Gold Chain, Golden Moss, Jack of the Buttery, Mousetail, Prick Madam, Stonecrop, Wall Ginger, Wallpepper

Botanical Name:
Sedum acre

Common Uses:

Eczema, Wound Care

Traditional Uses:
Stonecrop is traditionally used in ointments or applied directly to the skin to help ease pain and speed healing of burns, eczema, hemorrhoids, wounds, and ulcers and to aid in the removal of warts.

Parts Used:
Leaf, Stem

Side Effects:
Stonecrop is not recommended for use by women who are pregnant or nursing.

Stonecrop may cause skin irritation or blistering in some people.

Additional uses and side effects may exist but further research is necessary to determine the exact properties and effects of use.

General:
Stonecrop can be found throughout the Northern Hemisphere where it grows wild and is cultivated as an ornamental. The leaves are eaten as a raw or cooked vegetable and the leaf and stem are harvested for use fresh or as a tincture.

Sunflower
Adityabhakt, Corono Solis, Marigold of Peru, Sunflower

Botanical Name:
Helianthus annuus

Common Uses:
Natural Hair & Skin Care

Traditional Use:
Sunflower seed oil is an excellent source of Vitamin E and is used in natural cosmetic recipes to help combat wrinkles, promote a radiant glow, and to protect the hair & skin from UV rays and sun damage.

Part Used:
Leaf, Oil, Seed

Side Effects:
Sunflower is not recommended for use beyond dietary by women who are pregnant or nursing.

Sunflower may cause an allergic reaction in some people.

Sunflower may increase blood sugars.

Additional uses and side effects may exist but further research is necessary to determine the exact properties and effects of use.

General:

Sunflower is native to North America and is cultivated worldwide where the seeds are harvested for use as dietary oil or for use in supplement preparations. A traditional therapeutic dose of the oils in treating respiratory ailments is 15 drops 3 times daily. The leaves are harvested and dried for use as an infusion supplement.

Tamanu
Alexandrian Laurel, Indian Laurel, Kamani Punna, Palo Maria, Tamanu

Botanical Name:
Calophyllum inophyllum

Common Uses:
Acne, Eczema, Natural Skin Care, Psoriasis, Wound Care

Traditional Use:
Tamanu oil is rich oil with anti-inflammatory properties that is traditionally used in topical preparations to sooth symptoms and speed healing in conditions like acne, eczema, skin irritation, psoriasis, and wounds.

Tamanu oil is traditionally used to reduce scarring including acne scars, stretch marks.

Tamanu oil has been used as a traditional topical ointment or wash to speed healing of diabetic sores, fissures, chemical burns and herpes lesions.

Tamanu oil has significant antibacterial, antifungal, and antimicrobial qualities that make it a traditional treatment for a variety of infections like athlete's foot and staphylococcus.

Part Used:
Seed Oil

Side Effects:
Tamanu Oil is not recommended for use by women who are pregnant or nursing.

Tamanu Oil may cause dizziness, headache, and nausea.

General:
Tamanu is native to Africa, Asia and Australia but has been naturalized to other parts of the world as a fragrant ornamental. The seeds are harvested and the oils extracted by steam distillation for use in traditional topical and supplement preparations.

Tamarind
Imlee, Tamarind, Tintiri

Botanical Name:
Tamarindus indica

Common Uses:
Natural Skin Care, Wound Care

Traditional Use:
Tamarind oils have traditionally been used in natural skin care products as a tissue regeneration aide.

Tamarind has been used as a traditional poultice, ointment, or wash to reduce inflammation & infection while speeding healing in skin sores, ulcers, and wounds.

Part Used:
Fruit, Seed

Side Effects:
Tamarind is not recommended for use by women who are pregnant or nursing.

Additional uses and side effects may exist but further research is necessary to determine the exact properties and effects of use.

General:
Tamarind is a large evergreen native to Africa and has been naturalized to North & South America where the fruit is harvested when ripe for use as a food. The oil is extracted from the seed through steam distillation for use in topical preparations, cosmetics, and supplements.

Tarragon
Little Dragon, Mugwort, Tarragon

Botanical Name:
Artemisia dracunculus

Common Uses:
Contact Dermatitis

Traditional Use:
Tarragon has been used in traditional skin washes or ointments to reduce seepage and speed healing in skin sores, ulcers, and contact dermatitis pustules.

Part Used:
Leaf

Side Effects:
Tarragon is not recommended for use by women who are pregnant or nursing.

Tarragon is not recommended for long term use.

Tarragon may cause an allergic reaction in some people.

General:
Tarragon is native to Germany, Russia, and Southern Europe but is cultivated in many regions of the world where the leaves are harvested when in bloom, air dried, and used for culinary and supplement purposes or the oils are extracted through steam distillation for use in topical and aromatherapy preparations.

Tea

Black Tea, Chinese Tea, English Tea, Green Tea, Tea

Botanical Name:
Camellia sinensis

Common Uses:
Eczema, Natural Skin Care - Skin Irritation

Traditional Use:
Brown tea has traditionally been used to reduce the number and severity of eczema outbreaks. Studies indicate that drinking 4 or more cups of oolong tea per day may help to reduce eczema.

Tea has analgesic, astringent, and stimulant properties that make it a nice additive in washes and ointments designed to treat sensitive, irritated, or problem skin and is traditionally used to provide faster healing of bruises, varicose veins, skin eruptions, and sun burns.

Part Used:
Leaves

Side Effects:
Tea is not recommended for use in women who are pregnant or nursing.

Tea is not recommended for use by people who have anemia, anxiety, bleeding disorders, diabetes, glaucoma, heart problems, high blood pressure, or osteoporosis.

Tea is not recommended for use in women who have a hormone sensitive condition like endometriosis, fibroids, and cancer.

Overdose of tea may cause confusion, convulsions, diarrhea, dizziness, headache, heartburn, irregular heartbeat, nervousness, sleep problems, tremor, and vomiting.

Green tea contains compounds that may make anti-coagulant drugs less effective.

Tea does contain caffeine and overuse may lead to anxiety, frequent urination, irritability, insomnia, restlessness, and upset stomach.

There have been reports of liver problems in some people taking a concentrated tea extract over an extended period of time.

Tea may be addictive.

Additional uses and side effects may exist but further research is necessary to determine the exact properties and effects of use.

General:

Black, brown and green teas come from the same plant and the difference in coloring is a result of a change in the way that the tea is handled during processing. The more extensive handling of black tea changes its phytochemicals make up making the green tea the more beneficial supplement. Brown Tea is only partially fermented while Black Tea is fully fermented and Green Tea is not fermented. Tea is typically brewed and consumed as a beverage but is available in extract form. Therapeutic doses are traditionally believed to be reached by drinking 1 teaspoon of green tea leaf in 1 cup boiling water 5 times or more daily.

Teazle

Barber's Brush, Brushes & Combs, Card Thistle, Church Broom, Teazle

Botanical Name:
Dipsacus silvestris

Common Uses:
Eczema, Psoriasis, Wound Care

Traditional Use:
Teazle has traditionally been included in topical ointments for the treatment of eczema, fissures, psoriasis, and wound care.

Part Used:
Root, Whole

Side Effects:
Teazle is not recommended for use by women who are pregnant or nursing.

Additional uses and side effects may exist but further research is necessary to determine the exact properties and effects of use.

General:
Teazle grows wild in much of Africa, Asia, and Europe where it is harvested and processed as an extract. Teazle has long been used as a topical and supplement treatment but its actions and uses are not clearly defined.

Thyme

French Thyme, Garden Thyme, Red Thyme, Rubbed Thyme, Spanish Thyme, Thyme, Tomillo, Van Ajwayan, White Thyme

Botanical Name:
Thymus vulgaris

Common Uses:
Acne, Wound Care

Traditional Use:
Thyme tea is often included in topical preparations to reduce the severity of acne outbreaks.

Part Used:
Flower, Leaf, Stem

Side Effects:
Thyme is not recommended for use by women who are pregnant or nursing.

Thyme can cause an allergic reaction in some people.

Thyme oil may elevate the blood pressure.

Overuse of thyme can effect the menstrual cycles in some women

The oils isolated from the plant can be toxic and should not be ingested but the herb itself is generally considered safe.

Additional uses and side effects may exist but further research is necessary to determine the exact properties and effects of use.

General:
Thyme is native to the Mediterranean but is cultivated in many areas of the world where it is harvested as a culinary seasoning and as a liquid extract for use in traditional supplements. The oils are extracted through steam distillation for use in aromatherapy. Red Thyme and White Thyme oil come from the same plant. The alteration in coloring is due to oxidation during the extraction and processing of the oils. Red Thyme oil contains stronger anti-septic properties and is traditionally used for disinfection. White Thyme oil has more of the impurities removed and tends to have a milder action making it preferred in many traditional treatments.

Tribulus
Caltrop, Cat's Head, Devil's Thorn, Devil's Weed, Gouthead, Puncture Weed, Tribulus

Botanical Name:
Tribulus terrestris

Common Uses:
Eczema

Traditional Use:
Tribulus extracts are traditionally used to reduce the number and severity of certain types of eczema occurrences.

Part Used:
Fruit, Leaf, Seed

Side Effects:
Tribulus is not recommended for use by women who are pregnant or nursing.

Tribulus is not recommended for use by people who are taking nitroglycerine or have a heart condition.

Tribulus may act on the hormones and is not recommended for use by men who have prostate problems.

Tribulus may affect blood sugar levels.

The fruit of the Tribulus is not for internal use.

Additional uses and side effects may exist but further research is necessary to determine the exact properties and effects of use.

General:
Tribulus is native to India and has been naturalized to Africa, Asia, Central America, Europe, and North America where it is considered an invasive weed by some. The whole plant is harvested, dried, and powdered for use as a traditional supplement.

Turmeric
Curcuma, Halada, Haldi, Haridra, Indian Saffron, Nisha, Rajani, Turmeric, Yu Jin

Botanical Name:
Curcuma longa, Curcuma zedoaria

Common Uses:
Natural Skin Care, Wound Care

Traditional Use:
Turmeric supplements are used as a traditional supplement believed to work from the inside to help give skin a healthier, radiant glow.

Turmeric has traditionally been used to reduce the potential for infection in skin wounds & sores.

Part Used:
Rhizome, Underground Stems

Side Effects:
Turmeric is not recommended for use by women who are pregnant or nursing.

Turmeric may affect sugar levels do not use if you suffer from hyperglycemia or hypoglycemia.

Long term use or overdose of Turmeric may cause diarrhea, indigestion, or nausea in some people.

Turmeric is not for use by those with gall bladder disease.

Additional uses and side effects may exist but further research is necessary to determine the exact properties and effects of use.

General:
Turmeric is a shrub native to India and cultivated in China requiring warm temperatures and heavy moisture to survive. Turmeric is used in commercial and

traditional supplements as a tea, powder, or liquid extract or made into a powder for topical applications.

Vanilla
Botanical Name:
Vanilla planifolia

Common Uses:
Natural Skin Care

Traditional Use:
Vanilla oil has been included in natural skin care treatments for its softening and smoothing action.

Part Used:
Bean

Side Effects:
Vanilla is not recommended for use beyond dietary by women who are pregnant or nursing.

Vanilla may cause skin irritation, headache and insomnia.

Additional uses and side effects may exist but further research is necessary to determine the exact properties and effects of use.

General:
Vanilla is commonly used as a flavoring around the world but has also been used in traditional supplements and aromatherapy treatments.

Violet
Sweet Violet, Viola, Violet, Wild Violet

Botanical Name:
Viola oderata

Common Uses:
Natural Skin Care, Wound Care

Traditional Use:
Violet is used in natural skin care preparations to sooth the skin, ease dryness, and leave a silky feeling.

Violet leaves have been used in traditional poultices and washes to reduce pain & inflammation while minimizing infection in wounds.

Part Used:
Whole

Side Effects:
Violet is not recommended for use by women who are pregnant or nursing.

Violet contains aspirin-like compounds and is not recommended for use by those who have sensitivity to aspirin, have a bleeding disorder, are on blood thinning medications, or in children's treatments.

Additional uses and side effects may exist but further research is necessary to determine the exact properties and effects of use.

General:
Violet is cultivated throughout the world and is most common within the Northern Hemisphere. Violet buds & leaves are eaten as a raw or cooked vegetable or as a flavorful thickening agent in soups & desserts. Violet leaf oil is extracted for use in perfumery and in aromatherapy treatments. The whole plant is harvested during flowering, and used fresh or dried & powdered for use in traditional infusions and supplements.

Walnut
Akschota, English Walnut, He Tao, Juglands, Juglandis, Nogal, Walnussblatter, Walnut

Botanical Name:
Juglans

Common Uses:
Acne, Eczema, Natural Hair & Skin Care, Skin Inflammation

Traditional Uses:
Walnut leaf is traditionally applied directly or included in topical ointments & washes to reduce inflammation, stop seepage, and speed healing in skin conditions like acne, eczema, inflammation, and ulcers.

Walnut hulls yield a dark brownish black dye colorant and are traditionally used to dye fabrics, as hair colorant, or as part of sunless tanning lotions.

Parts Used:
Nut, Shell – Hull

Side Effects:
Walnut is not recommended for use beyond dietary for women who are pregnant or nursing.

Walnut may cause softening of the stools, bloating and weight gain if it is used in excess.

Additional uses and side effects may exist but further research is necessary to determine the exact properties and effects of use.

General:
Walnut is the seed of the trees in the Jugulans family. Walnuts are eaten as a food and the nuts & hulls are used as a traditional supplement, cosmetic, and colorant.

Watercress
Agriao, Berros, Cresson, Indian Cress, Nasilord, Scruvy Grass, Tall Nasturtium, Watercress

Botanical Name:
Nasturtium officinale

Common Uses:
Acne

Traditional Use:
Watercress juice has been used as a traditional facial wash to reduce acne blemishes.

Part Used:
Whole

Side Effects:
Watercress is not recommended for women who are pregnant or nursing.

Watercress is not recommended for children.

Watercress may cause gastrointestinal upset including flatulence and nausea.

Additional uses and side effects may exist but further research is necessary to determine the exact properties and effects of use.

General:
Watercress is found in nearly every region of the world where it is harvested during the flowering season for use in salads or as a traditional supplement tea up to 4 times daily before meals.

Wheat
Botanical Name:
Triticum aestivum

Common Uses:
Contact Dermatitis, Damaged Skin, Eczema, Irritated Skin, Psoriasis

Traditional Use:
Wheat is traditionally added to baths & scrub bags to help alleviate itching associated with contact dermatitis, eczema, and psoriasis and to help heal damaged skin.

Side Effects:
Wheat is not recommended for use by women who are pregnant or nursing.

Additional uses and side effects may exist but further research is necessary to determine the exact properties and effects of use.

General:
Wheat is cultivated as a food crop in Asia, Europe and North America. Wheat is also used as a traditional supplement or topical preparation up to 2 times daily.

White Nettle
Archangel, Bee Nettle, Blind Nettle, Deaf Nettle, Dumb Nettle, Stingless Nettle, White Nettle

Botanical Name:
Lamium album

Common Uses:
Contact Dermatitis, Skin Irritation & Inflammation

Traditional Use:
White Nettles have been incorporated into traditional washes to help alleviate skin irritation from contact dermatitis.

Part Used:
Flower, Leaf

Side Effects:
White Nettle is not recommended for use by women who are pregnant or nursing.

Additional uses and side effects may exist but further research is necessary to determine the exact properties and effects of use.

General:
White Nettle is native in Asia and Europe where the leaves are eaten as a raw or cooked vegetable. The flower and leaf have been harvested, dried, and powdered for use in traditional supplement teas up to 3 times daily and for use as a topical poultice or wash.

Witch Hazel
Botanical Name:
Hamamelis virginiana

Common Uses:
Acne, Eczema, Natural Hair & Skin Care, Skin Rash, Psoriasis, Wound Care

Traditional Use:
The bark oil of witch hazel is combined with an alcohol base to create a soothing, astringent wash that works to sooth a variety of skin conditions from acne and eczema to varicose veins and eye puffiness.

Part Used:
Bark, Leaf, Oil

Side Effects:
Witch Hazel is not recommended for internal use by women who are pregnant or nursing.

Witch Hazel is not recommended for internal use. Internal use may cause constipation, gastrointestinal upset, liver problems and other side effects.

Additional uses and side effects may exist but further research is necessary to determine the exact properties and effects of use.

General:
Hamamelis virginiana is a species of Witch Hazel that is native to North America. The bark is harvested and distilled for use in traditional supplements, topical preparations, and commercial products.

Woad

Ben Lan Gen, Chinese Indigo, Dyer's Woad, Farberwaid, Glastum, Hierba Pastel, Indigo Woad, Isatis, Quing Dai, Woad

Botanical Name:
Isatis tinctoria

Common Uses:
Psoriasis

Traditional Use:
Woad has traditionally been used in topical preparations to help alleviate psoriasis.

Part Used:
Leaf, Root

Side Effects:
Woad is not recommended for use by women who are pregnant or nursing.

Woad is not recommended for use in children's treatments.

Woad contains aspirin like substances and is not recommended for use by people with an allergy to asthma.

Woad is not recommended for people on blood thinning medication.

Additional uses and side effects may exist but further research is necessary to determine the exact properties and effects of use.

General:
Woad is native to Asia but is naturalized to Europe and North America where it has been cultivated as a blue dye product for thousands of years. The leaf and root are harvested for use fresh or dried in traditional supplements. Alcohol extracts are undergoing study as a potential treatment for slowing the growth of cancer cells.

Yarrow

Achilee, Milfoil, Nosebleed, Old Man's Pepper, Soldier's Woundwort, Staunchweed, Yarrow

Botanical Name:
Achillea millefolium

Common Uses:
Acne, Eczema, Scars, Wound Care

Traditional Use:
Yarrow has been used as a topical preparation to cleanse the skin and reduce the severity of acne outbreaks while also being taken as a supplement to cleanse the body of impurities helping to limit the number and severity of future outbreaks.

Yarrow is traditionally used to help heal inflamed cuts and wounds while minimizing scarring and soothing chronic conditions like eczema.

Part Used:
Flower, Leaf, Oil, Stem

Side Effects:
Yarrow is believed to have an abortifacient effect and is not recommended for use by women who are pregnant or nursing.

Yarrow may cause photosensitivity, allergic reactions, or skin irritation.

Yarrow is intended for short term use only.

Overuse of Yarrow can be toxic.

Overuse of Yarrow may cause headaches & dizziness.

General:
Yarrow is native to Asia and Europe and has been naturalized to North America growing wild in dry fields and untended areas. Yarrow is harvested, dried, and powdered for use in traditional supplement infusions given up to 4 times daily.

Yellow Dock

Acedera, Amalvelas, Broad Leaved Dock, Curled Dock, Field Sorrel, Narrow Dock, Rumex, Sheep Sorrel, Sour Dock, Yellow Dock

Botanical Name:
Rumex crispus

Common Uses:
Acne, Contact Dermatitis, Eczema, Skin Irritation, Poison Ivy, Psoriasis,

Traditional Use:
Yellow dock tea has traditionally been used as a supplement to help detoxify the body and treat chronic skin conditions and has also been incorporated into a wash to aid in reducing certain types of acne, eczema, psoriasis, and itchy contact dermatitis including poison ivy.

Part Used:
Root

Side Effects:
Yellow Dock is not recommended for use by women who are pregnant or nursing.

Overuse of Yellow Dock may cause potassium depletion.

Overuse of Yellow Dock may cause cramps, diarrhea, excessive urination, nausea, and skin irritation.

Overuse of Yellow Dock may irritate the mucus membranes and should not be used by people with ulcers.

Yellow dock may cause or aggravate kidney stones.

Yellow Dock may cause allergies in some people.

Yellow Dock may speed clotting.

Additional uses and side effects may exist but further research is necessary to determine the exact properties and effects of use.

General:
Yellow dock is native to Africa and Europe but has naturalized to other areas including the United States where some consider it an invasive weed. Yellow Dock prefers high moisture, porous soil and plenty of sunlight for optimal growth. The leaf is used as a salad food and the root is harvested in the spring, dried and powdered for use in traditional supplement teas and topical preparations.

Appendix B – Glossary

Abortifacient – is a substance that is capable of inducing an abortion

Adoptogenic – is a substance that has a normalize effect against changes brought about by stressors

Alopecia – A condition where hair is lost or partially lost from a place where it normally grows also called baldness.

Amenorrhea – refers to the absence of normal menstruation.

Analgesic - is a pain-killing drug or medicine.

Anodyne - is a pain-killing drug or medicine.

Antibacterial – is a substance that is active against bacteria.

Anti-Convulsant – is a substance used to reduce or prevent convulsions.

Anti-Emetic – is a substance that reduces or prevents nausea or vomiting.

Anti-Fungal – is a substance that alleviates or prevents fungal infections.

Antihistamine - is a substance that inhibits the physiological effects of histamine. Histamine is the chemical released by the body during an allergic reaction.

Anti-Inflammatory – is a substance used to reduce inflammation.

Anti-Microbial- is a substance that kills or inhibits the growth of microorganisms

Anti-Oxidant – is a molecule that inhibits the oxidation of other molecules.

Anti-Periodic – is a substance used to treat malarial-type symptoms or to prevent the recurrence of malarial like symptoms.

Anti-Parasitic – is a substance used to treat or prevent parasitic infestations.

Anti-Septic – is a substance capable of preventing or treating infection by inhibiting the growth of microorganisms.

Anti-Spasmodic - is a substance that suppresses muscle spasms.

Anti-Tussive – is a substance used to suppress or relieve coughing.

Anti-Viral – is a substance that prevents or treats viral infections by killing a virus or that suppresses its ability to replicate.

Aphrodisiac – is a substance that stimulates sexual desire.

Aromatic – is a substance having a pleasant and distinctive smell that is used as a treatment.

Aroma Therapy – is the process of using an aromatic plant extract or essential oil to cause a physical or psychological effect in treatments.

Aspergillus - is a type of common mold that cause food spoilage and potentially disease.

Astringent - is a substance that causes the contraction of body tissues.

Botanical Name – is the Latin name give to a species of plant to distinguish it from other plants.

Bursitis – is a condition where there is inflammation in the bursa – elbow, knee, shoulder.

Cardiac – refers to the heart.

Carminative – is a substance that relieves flatulence.

Cathartic - is a purgative substance.

Chalagogue - is a substance that stimulates the secretion of bile from the gallbladder.

Coagulant - is a substance that causes blood to clot or coagulate

Colorant - is a substance that colors something usually food, cosmetics, or textile products.

Common Name – is the non-specific name used for everyday reference to a plant

Comminution – is the action of reducing a material or substance. When processing plants the act of reducing the size of the plant parts by cutting, grinding, or pounding

Conjunctivitis – is an infection or irritation causing inflammation, itching, and redness of the white part of the eye.

COPD – stands for Chronic Obstructive Pulmonary Disease, which is a disorder that involves constriction of the airways and difficulty breathing.

Decoction – is the result of concentration the essence of a substance or plant part by heating or boiling.

Demulcent – is a substance that soothes inflammation and protects irritated internal tissues.

Depurative – is a substance that facilitates the removal of impurities or cleansing of bodily fluids.

Detoxification - is the process of removing toxic substances or qualities from matter.

Diaphoretic – is a substance that induces perspiration.

Diosgenin – is a steroid compound used in the synthesis of steroid hormones.

Diuretic – is a substance causing increased passing of urine.

Dram – is a unit of measurement equaling approximately 1/16 of a dry weight ounce in US measurement 1/8 of a fluid ounce in Apothecary measurement.

Dysmenorrheal – refers to menstruation with excessive pain involving abdominal and lower back cramping.

Emetic - is a substance that causes vomiting.

Emmenagogue – is a substance that stimulates or increases menstrual flow.

Emollient – is a substance that has a softening or soothing affect on the skin.

Estrogenic – is a substance acting like, relating to, or caused by estrogen.

Expectorant – is a substance that promotes the secretion of mucus from the air passages.

Expression – is the process of forcibly separating liquids from solids.

Febrifuge – is a substance used to reduce fever.

Fluid extract – is a type of fluid-solid substance obtained from plant matter through water or alcohol processing

Galactogogue - is a substance that stimulates milk secretion.

Glycosides – is a compound formed from a simple sugar and another compound by the replacement of a hydroxyl in the sugar molecules.

Gram-Positive Bacteria – is a class of bacterial that are stained dark blue or violet by gram staining including bacteria such as pneumococci, staphylococci, and streptococci.

Gram Negative Bacteria - A class of bacterial that do not retain the stain used in gram staining including bacteria such as e. coli, shingella, and salmonella.

Hallucinogenic – is a psychoactive substance capable of producing hallucinations or altered sensory experiences.

Hepatic – refers to being of or relating to the liver.

Hydration – is the process of combining with or giving water.

Hypoallergenic – is a substance unlikely to cause an allergic reaction.

Hypoglycemic – is a condition indicated by low blood sugar.

Hypotensive – is a condition of abnormally low blood pressure.

Histamine – is the chemical released by the body during an allergic reaction.

Immuno-Stimulant - is a substance that stimulates the immune system to fight infection.

Infusion – Aqueous – is a drink or extract made by soaking plant parts in water.

Infusion – Oil – is a drink, extract, or product made by soaking plant parts in oil.

Insecticide - Substance used for killing insects.

Interferon - is a protein released in response to a virus that has the ability to inhibit virus reproduction.

Laxative – is a substance that stimulates or facilitates evacuation of the bowels

Lipase – is an enzyme that facilitates the breakdown of fats to fatty acids and glycol to other alcohols.

Maceration – is the process of softening plant materials by soaking or steeping in a liquid. To separate the compounds by soaking or steeping

Menorrhagia – refers to abnormally heavy menstrual bleeding.

Menstruum - is a solvent or mix of solvents.

Microphage – is a cell found in the tissues or at the site of an infection that takes in foreign material.

Mordant – is a substance that combines with a dye or stain to fix the colorant into a material.

Muscle Relaxant – is a substance that reduces muscle tone or contractibility.

Narcotic – is a psychoactive substance affecting mood or behavior.

Nervine – is a psychoactive substance that calms the nerves.

Nutritive – is a substance that is nutritious or provides nourishment.

Percolation – is the extraction of soluble components by passing the liquid through a filtering medium.

Pharynx – is the membrane-lined cavity behind the nose and mouth that connects them to the esophagus.

Phytoestrogen – are compounds found in plants that can mimic the effects of estrogen.

Pleurae – is the membranes lining the thorax and enveloping the lungs.

Pleurisy – is an inflammation of the pleurae that causes pain when breathing.

Polysaccharide – is a carbohydrate that is a compound of sugar molecules bonded together.

Proof Spirit – is a mixture of alcohol and water containing 50% alcohol by volume standard in the US.

Purgative – is a substance that is strongly laxative in effect.

Pulmonary – relates to the pulmonary system.

Phytosterol – is a group of naturally occurring steroid plant compounds.

Reparative – is a substance that helps to repair.

Rhinitis – is the inflammation of the mucus membrane of the nose.

Rubefacient – is a substance whose external application produces increased circulation or redness of the skin.

Saponins – is a class of steroid and terpenoid glycosides that are used in detergents and foams when shaken with water.

Sciatica – refers to nerve pain caused by compression of a spinal nerve in the lower back that affects the back, hip, or leg.

Sedative – is a substance that causes a calming or sleep-inducing effect.

Squalene – is an oily liquid that is the precursor to sterols.

Sterols – is a naturally occurring unsaturated steroid alcohol.

Steroidal – relates to steroid hormones or their effects.

Stimulant – is a substance that raises levels of physiological or nervous activity in the body.

Styptic – is a substance that causes bleeding to stop.

Succus – refers to several liquids in the body commonly termed digestive juices but also to the juice of fresh plant material.

Tincture – is a substance made by dissolving plant materials in alcohol.

Vasodilator – is a substance that causes dilation of blood vessels.

Vermifuge – is a substance that destroys parasites.

Viscosity – is the resistance of a liquid to movement and flow.

www.ingramcontent.com/pod-product-compliance
Lightning Source LLC
Chambersburg PA
CBHW082133290526
45794CB00008B/3016